ALSO BY JANICE COX

Natural Beauty from the Garden

Natural Beauty for All Seasons

Natural Beauty at Home

SECOND EDITION

Natural Beauty at Home

MORE THAN 250 EASY-TO-USE RECIPES
FOR BODY, BATH, AND HAIR

Janice Cox

Illustrated by Dorothy Reinhardt

An Owl Book
Henry Holt and Company / New York

I DEDICATE THIS BOOK TO MY FAMILY

*my wonderful and supportive husband, Ray,
and my two natural beauties, Lauren and Marie.*

Henry Holt and Company, LLC
Publishers since 1866
*115 West 18th Street
New York, New York 10011*

*Henry Holt ® is a registered trademark of
Henry Holt and Company, LLC.*

Library of Congress Cataloging-in-Publication Data
Cox, Janice.
   *Natural beauty at home : more than 250 easy-to-use recipes for body, bath,
and hair / Janice Cox ; illustrated by Dorothy Reinhardt. — 2nd ed.*
      p.   cm.
   "An owl book."
   Includes index.
   ISBN 0-8050-7022-2 (pbk.)
   1. Beauty, Personal.   2. Skin—Care and hygiene.   3. Hair—Care
and hygiene. 4. Herbal cosmetics.   I. Title.
RA778 .C755 2002
646.7'2—dc21   2001051757

*Henry Holt books are available for special promotions and
premiums. For details contact: Director, Special Markets.*

*First Edition 1995
Second Edition 2002*

DESIGNED BY LUCY ALBANESE

Printed in the United States of America

5   7   9   10   8   6

Acknowledgments

I want to thank the outstanding team of people that helped me revise and produce this new book.

To all my dear friends, family members, and readers who share my passion for "home beauty," your feedback and ideas are invaluable to me.

To my agent, Laurie Harper: Thank you for your enthusiasm for my work; you are awesome.

To my editor at Henry Holt, Deborah Brody: Thank you for your direction and insight in improving my original book and making it even better.

Also, I thank Rebecca Lindenberg for all of her efforts that helped make this book easy to revise and edit.

A special thank-you to Darlene Barbaria for a stunning cover design, Nora Reichard for her thorough job of copyediting, Dorothy Reinhardt for her original artwork, and Kristin Minnick for her publicity work. You are all the best.

A final thank-you to everyone at Henry Holt for their time and effort; it makes my job pure pleasure. You all deserve a bit of pampering—you are all beautiful!

Note

The recipes and treatments contained in this book are generally safe and effective. However, despite every effort to offer expert advice it is not possible for this book to predict an individual person's reactions to a particular recipe or treatment. The reader should consult a qualified physician. Neither the publisher, Henry Holt and Company, nor the author, Janice Cox, accepts responsibility for any effects that may arise from following the recipes or treatments and using the products from the recipes in this book.

Contents

Introduction *1*

Five Factors That Can Affect Your Skin and Hair *6* • A Note About the Recipes *7*

Equipment and Ingredients *9*

Beauty Shopping *13* • Basic Natural Beauty Ingredients *15* • Substitutions *25* • Beauty Tools from Nature *26* • Weights and Measures *28* • Metric Equivalents *28*

Cleansers and Scrubs *29*

Natural Soap Alternatives *32* • Oatmeal Cleanser *33* • Cleansing Milk *33* • Empress Josephine's Cleanser *34* • All-Purpose Honey Cleanser *34* • Olive Oil Cleansing Lotion *35* • Arrowroot Cleansing Jelly *35* • Strawberry Cleanser *36* • Grapefruit Cleanser *36* • Country Fresh Dairy Cleanser *37* • Gentle Eye Makeup Remover *37* • Almond Cleansing Scrub *38* • Favorite Cleansing Grains *38* • Orange Peel Scrub *39* • Avocado

Stone Scrub *40* • Apricot Kernel Scrub *41* • Sublime Sunflower Scrub *42* • Sugar Scrub *43* • Oatmeal Elbow Cream *43* • Pumice Scrub for the Feet *44*

Astringents, Toners, and Skin Fresheners 45

Basic Astringent *48* • Astringent for Sensitive Skin *48* • Apple Juice Astringent *49* • Strawberry Leaf Astringent *49* • Orange-Mint Toner *50* • Honey Toner *51* • Cooling Cucumber Toner *51* • Mint-Vinegar Toner *52* • Fennel Seed and Honey Toner *52* • Green Tea Skin Toner *53* • Vitamin C Toner *54* • Citrus Freshener *55* • Chamomile Skin Freshener *55* • Gin Skin Tonic *56* • Lavender Freshener *57* • Beauty Water *57* • One-Minute Skin Type Test *58*

Creams and Lotions 59

Basic Cold Cream *63* • Original Greek Cold Cream *64* • California Cold Cream *65* • Cucumber Cold Cream *66* • Almond Oil Lotion *67* • Australian Frangipani Lotion *68* • Lecithin Moisturizer *69* • Australian Lanolin Cream *70* • Basic Moisturizer *71* • Coconut Cloud Cream *72* • Corn Flour Lotion *73* • Body Butter *73* • Grape Seed Oil Lotion *74* • Papaya Cream *75* • Refreshing Leg Gel *76* • Health Nut Lotion *76* • Floral Aloe Vera Gel *77* • Cooling Aloe Lotion *78* • Witch Hazel Body Lotion *78* • Allover Nighttime Lotion *79* • Alligator Pear Lotion *80* • Super Eye Cream *81* • Firming Neck Cream *82* • Tropical Eye Cream *82* • Yarrow Lotion *83* • Mint Body Lotion *84* • Mermaid Lotion *85* • Stretch Mark Cream *86* • Rose Lotion *87*

Facial Treatments 89

Give Yourself a Great Facial *93* • Beauty Mayo *94* • Marie Antoinette Mask *95* • Apricot Facial Mask *96* • Country Garden Facial Mask *96* •

Surprise-Party Facial Mask *97* • Old-Fashioned Oatmeal Masks *98* •
Beauty Queen Mask *99* • Natural Clay Masks *99* • Salsa Facial *101* •
Summer Watermelon Mask *101* • Mediterranean Mask *102* • Swiss Milk-
maid Mask *102* • Swedish Rose Hip Mask *103* • Brewer's Yeast Mask
104 • Fruit Gel Masks *105* • Single-Ingredient Masks from Nature's Skin
Salon *106* • Piña Colada Mask *107* • Strawberry Acne Mask *108* • Fresh
Carrot Mask *108* • Acne or Troubled-Skin Care *109* • Natural Eye Care
110 • Cooling Eye Gel *111*

Lip Treatments *113*

Aloe Vera Lip Gloss *116* • Almond and Cocoa Butter Lip Gloss *116* • Flavored Coconut Lip Gloss *117* • Coconut-Almond Lip Gloss *117* • Vanilla
Lip Gloss *118* • Chocolate Lip Gloss *118* • Castor Oil Lip Balm *119* •
Beeswax Lipsticks *119* • Lip Stains *120* • Chapped Lip Cure *121* • Luscious Lips *122*

Hydrotherapy: Shower and Bath Treatments *123*

Morning Wake-up! *126* • Pineapple Body Seltzer *126* • Vinegar-Herb
Bath *127* • Cleopatra Milk Bath *128* • Super Muscle-Soothing Bath *129*
• Herb Baths *129* • Northwest Pine Bath *130* • Rose Floral Bath *131* •
Oatmeal Cookie Bath *132* • Colored Bath Salts *132* • Old-Fashioned Bub-
ble Bath *133* • Scrubbing Sacks *134* • Fizzing Bath Bombs *135* • Mus-
tard Bath *136* • Foaming Bath Salts *136* • Relaxing Lavender Bath *137*
• Creating the Ultimate Bath Environment *138*

Body Treatments *139*

Salt Rub *142* • Raw Sugar Scrub *143* • Exfoliation *144* • Herbal Body
Wrap *145* • Sea Mud Body Mask *145* • Thalassotherapy *146* • Tropi-
cal Body Polish *147* • Yogurt Body Treatment *147* • Dry Brushing *148*
• English Ivy Body Massage *149* • Green Goddess Body Mask *151* •

Loofah Body Polish *152* • Mehndi-Henna Tattoos *152* • Sun Sense *154* • Sunburn Soothers *155*

Massage Oils and Aromatherapy *157*

How to Give a Great Massage *160* • Amorous Massage Oil *161* • Herb Massage Oil *162* • Hot Rock Massage *163* • Citrus Massage Oil *163* • Sore Muscle Massage Oil *164* • Oil of Oils *164* • Gardenia Oil *165* • Cooling Massage Spirits *166* • Zanzibar Foot Oil *166* • Vintage Oil *167* • Natural Energy *168*

Hair-Care Products *169*

Shampoo Tips *171* • Basic Shampoo A *173* • Basic Shampoo B *173* • Herbal Shampoo *174* • Egg Shampoo *174* • Body and Bounce Beer Shampoo *175* • Desert Wonder Shampoo *175* • Sunshine Shampoo *176* • Olive Oil Shampoo *176* • Dry Shampoos *177* • Basil Shampoo Powder *178* • Rice Flour Dry Shampoo *178* • Conditioning Hair Packs *179* • Honey (Molasses) Hair Pack *180* • Perfect Hair Conditioner *181* • Rock Melon Hair Conditioner *181* • Roaring Twenties Conditioner *182* • Tucson Jojoba Oil and Beer Conditioner *182* • Caribbean Rum Conditioner *183* • Dandruff-Control Treatments *183* • Natural Hair Rinses *184* • Highlighting Hair Rinses *185* • Watercress Rinse for Oily Hair *186* • Dandruff Rinse *186* • Henna Hair Color *187* • Henna Enhancers *189* • Egyptian Henna Conditioning Treatment *190* • Basic Hair Gel *190* • Pink Grapefruit Styling Gel *191* • Almond Oil Hair Gel *192* • Champagne Hair Gel *193* • Brilliantine *193* • Rosemary Hair Oil *194* • Jalapeño Hair Tonic *194* • Lemon Hair Spray *195* • Psyllium-Seed Setting Lotion *196* • Sugar Hair Spray *196* • Swimming Pool Hair Care *197*

Nail Treatments *199*

Manicure for Healthy Hands and Nails *202* • Jojoba Nail and Cuticle Oil *204* • Cocoa Cuticle Cream *204* • Natural Nail Polish *205* • Molasses

Nail Soak *205* • Pineapple Cuticle Softener *206* • Evening Nail Oil *206* • Nail Hardener *207* • Henna Nail Treatment *207* • Castor Oil Nail Rub *208* • Nail Whitener *208* • Paraffin Hand Treatment *209*

Fragrance *211*

Effleurage 216 • Eau de Cologne 217 • Hungary Water 217 • Victorian Handkerchief Cologne 218 • Irresistible Rose Cologne 218 • Orchid Isle Cologne 219 • Summer Garden Cologne 220 • Mona Lisa Voile 220 • Lavender Dry Perfume 221 • Citrus Dry Perfume 222 • After-Bath Splash 222 • Attar of Roses 223 • Solid Perfume 224 • Lavender Linen Spray 224

Powders *225*

Chlorophyll *228* • Simple Bath Powder *228* • Scented Bath Powder *229* • Scented Rice Flour Powder *230* • Almond Oil Powder *231* • Peppermint Powder *232* • Orange-Flower Powder *233* • Rose Geranium Powder *234* • Violet Powder *234* • Deodorant Powder *235* • Carmen Miranda Fruit Powder *236* • Cloud Nine Powder *237* • Cooling Cinnamon Powder *238*

Mouthwashes and Tooth Powders *239*

Herb Garden Mouthwash *242* • Rose Water Mouthwash *242* • Clove Mouthwash *243* • Strawberry Leaf Mouth Rinse *243* • Natural Mouth Fresheners *244* • Salt Water Rinse *245* • Tooth Powders *245* • Soothing Tooth Powder *246* • Lavender Mouth Rinse *247* • Peppermint Toothpaste *247* • Healthy Smile *248*

Soap and Soap Making *249*

Soap-Making Equipment *252* • Basic Soap-Making Rules *253* • Ingredient Temperatures for Soap Making *253* • Tallow Soap *254* • Basic Castile

Soap *255* • Coconut Oil Soap *256* • Cold-Cream Soap *258* • Oatmeal Soap *259* • Glycerine Soap *260* • Super-Easy Oatmeal Soap *262* • Some Variations to Try in Soap Making *263* • Soap Treasures *264* • Easy Soap Balls *265* • Loofah Soap *266*

Antiperspirants and Deodorants **267**

Antiperspirant Spray *270* • Natural Deodorant Cream *270* • Botanical Deodorant *271* • Citrus Deodorant *271*

Products for Men **273**

Shaving Tips *275* • Bay Rum Aftershave *277* • Soothing Aftershave *277* • Old West Aftershave *278* • Roman Empire Aftershave *278* • Vitalizing Skin Bracer *279* • Electric Pre-shave *280* • Basic Shaving Cream *280* • Cleansing Facial Scrubs *281* • Almond Oil Shaving Cream *282* • Invigorating Foot Rub *282* • Athlete's-Foot Cure *283* • Pumice Hand Scrub *284* • Avocado Oil Hair Pack *284* • Horseradish Hair Treatment *285* • Moustache Wax *285* • Crew-Cut Oil *286*

Products for Children **287**

Baby Powder *290* • Baby Oil *291* • Baby Massage *291* • Coconut Baby Oil *293* • Diaper Cream *293* • New Baby Bath *294* • Honey Bee Bath *295* • Fresh Strawberry Bath *295* • Bubbles, Bubbles, Bubbles *296* • Have Fun! *296* • Sweet Dreams Bath *297* • Tutti-Frutti Lip Gloss *297* • Marie's Glitter Gloss *298* • Fantasy Face Paints *298* • Scented Play Dough *299*

Glossary of Terms **301**

Index **305**

Natural Beauty at Home

Introduction

*I*n 1994, I put together my personal collection of home beauty recipes and called it *Natural Beauty at Home.* My goal was to share my own passion with others, and I am so glad I did! This book has become a classic text for any natural beauty enthusiast.

Each year I get hundreds of letters and e-mails from readers who are enjoying the art of creating their own natural beauty products. Many of you have enjoyed saving money and looking and feeling better than ever before. Some of you have even started your own natural beauty businesses—selling fresh creams and potions using these easy-to-follow recipes. Hearing all these stories of clear skin, shiny hair, beauty parties, and new ingredient discoveries has been very rewarding and fun for me.

I, too, have changed. Natural beauty was always my hobby and passion, and now it is my career. With three books, hundreds of magazine articles, a website, and numerous radio and television appearances, I am happily spreading the word about natural beauty. When I was given the opportunity to revise and improve my original book, I could not resist the chance to give my readers more recipes, more beauty ideas, and more new treatments. I have added more than fifty new recipes, with Fizzing Bath Bombs, Green Tea Skin Toner, and Chocolate Lip Gloss being some of my new favorites. I have also updated several other recipes, adding easy-to-find ingredient substitutions or better formulas.

To think it all started back in junior high when I first experimented in my parents' bathroom with egg facials and oatmeal scrubs. I was looking for homemade alternatives to cosmetic products that I saw in my mother's magazines.

In high school and college, beauty treatments became a social affair for me. Somehow, facial masks, manicures, and pedicures seem more effective if done in a group. It is also a great time to discuss life and to take yourself less seriously. How can you with green avocado all over your face?

I studied chemistry in college and continue to be amazed by chemical reactions and how they relate to cosmetic products. Keeping oil and water mixed together into the perfect emulsion or moisturizer is not only fun but also fascinating.

Today my whole family has become a part of my natural beauty projects. My husband and two daughters often help me test new recipes. They are all very tolerant of all my potions and ingredients stored all over the house. I also love to travel, which has helped me in my search for new recipes and ingredients. I was thrilled to find wonderful macadamia oil in Hawaii, and a trip to Paris yielded many new formulas. The French are renowned for their beauty products and treatments, which are some of the best in the world. Beauty really is all around us, and one thing I have discovered over the years is when it comes to looking and feeling terrific the world really is a small place— people throughout the world enjoy doing something for themselves.

Many of the recipes in this book are ones I remember my grandmother and mother using. My mother was a home economics education major in college and is an excellent cook. She gave me a firm foundation in the kitchen and the confidence to tackle any recipe. My grandmother is also an excellent cook. I remember reading cookbooks at her house the way many people read novels. They also taught me many beauty basics. My mother's rule of never going to bed with a dirty face, and my grandmother's of counting to twenty when rinsing my face, have become a part of my everyday regime. In researching this book I found that many families have their own home beauty recipes and treatments. For example, my husband's grandmother made her own soap for the family, and his aunts make their own night creams and moisturizers.

Throughout history, cosmetics have played a role in shaping people's lives. The invention of soap alone is said to have added years to the average human life span by killing bacteria and thus reducing the amount of sickness and disease in the world. Homemade recipes of great beauties such as Cleopatra, Marie Antoinette, and Helen of Troy are scattered throughout history books.

Making your own beauty products is simple to do, cost-effective, and fun. Even though I occasionally purchase cosmetics, I find that my own recipes work just as well, if not better, than commercial brands because they are pure and undiluted. You control the ingredients used, and you know there is no cruel animal testing involved.

I have always focused on the enjoyment of making my own cosmetics, but I cannot ignore the cost savings. When you realize what you have been spending on commercial products and how much it costs to create your own homemade versions, you'll be amazed and delighted. The cost of these ingredients is nothing compared to what companies spend on packaging and marketing their products, which is reflected in their retail prices. You can purchase a honey toner from a well-known natural cosmetic manufacturer for sixteen dollars, or you can make the Honey Toner recipe on page 51 for around eighty-five cents—quite a difference! I once met a lady in her seventies who had worked her whole life for a major cosmetics firm. She told me I could do just as well spreading vegetable shortening on my face as using their most expensive night cream. Many women spend sixty to seventy dollars for expensive night and eye creams when they could make their own products for a few dollars.

Today you can't pass a cosmetic shop or display without seeing the word *natural.* All of a sudden, "back to basics" is a trend, and less is definitely better when it comes to beauty and beauty products. There are even natural beauty boutiques now where the products are so fresh you must rush home and pop them in the refrigerator and throw them out after a few days. *Commercial companies cannot make cosmetics fresher than you can at home.* Time works against them as they mass-produce their products and transport them to retail outlets. Commercial products are made to handle any possible problem that could arise before you purchase them. They are made to withstand a wide range of temperatures (from freezing to boiling) and have a very long shelf life.

This book contains some of my very favorite recipes and treatments and has been updated to include some of the more current trends in natural cosmetic products. The recipes are easy to follow and use ingredients that can be found in your local supermarket or natural food store. The recipes call for modern

TEN STEPS TO NATURAL BEAUTY

1. Get plenty of rest.
2. Exercise regularly.
3. Eat a balanced diet (the basic food pyramid).
4. Drink at least eight glasses of water daily.
5. Keep your skin and hair clean and nourished.
6. Give yourself a weekly facial and monthly total body treatment.
7. Brush your teeth after every meal.
8. Use sun protection.
9. Use natural beauty products.
10. Smile!

kitchen equipment such as a saucepan, measuring cups, and a blender—nothing exotic. Many of the procedures involve simply mixing together a few ingredients in the right proportions. None of the recipes requires any more skill than boiling water and being able to follow directions. Try one or all of the recipes, by yourself or with a friend. Once you've made your first cosmetic product, I know that, like me, you will be hooked.

Remember that we are all born with a natural beauty. It is how we choose to use it that makes us truly beautiful.

FIVE FACTORS THAT CAN AFFECT YOUR SKIN AND HAIR

Diet: Diet is probably the most important factor that affects the health of your skin and hair. It is just as important to feed and moisturize from within as from outside. A well-balanced diet with lots of fresh fruits, vegetables, and calcium—and plenty of water—will do more for your skin and hair than the most expensive cosmetics.

Medication: When taking medication, consult your physician if you see any changes in your skin and hair. Birth control pills and other hormonal medications can affect the skin, sometimes resulting in dry, flaky skin or rashes, as does tetracycline, a common antibiotic.

Environment: The environment can affect our skin and hair. Sun and wind are very drying and break down the collagen in our skin. Wind can chap the skin and dry out the hair. Smog can cover the skin and hair with a thin layer of dirt. Air-conditioning and indoor heating systems can also affect the health of our skin and hair. Always use sun protection, and keep your hair and skin clean and well moisturized.

Physical activity: Exercise is important for healthy skin and hair. Physical activity gets your blood flowing and does wonders for your complexion. It is also important to get plenty of rest. The average adult requires eight to nine hours of sleep each night, but few of us consistently get that much!

Heredity: Healthy skin and hair, as well as skin problems, can be passed down through the genes we inherit from our parents. Acne is a common skin problem that can be inherited. Proper skin and hair care can help to improve these conditions and even overcome them—so do not feel as if there is nothing you can do if these conditions run in your family.

A NOTE ABOUT THE RECIPES

The recipes contained in this book are 100 percent color-free and can be made fragrance-free. I have suggested different scents, but these are always optional ingredients. The color and scent of these products are derived from their own natural ingredients.

Preservatives are not needed in many of these recipes either because the ingredients act as a natural preservative or the recipe yields enough for only one application. When natural preservatives such as vitamin C or tincture of benzoin are suggested, these, too, can be optional. If you choose not to use a preservative, certain recipes may need refrigeration.

If you are sensitive to a known ingredient, either find a suitable substitute (olive oil rather than almond oil) or choose a different recipe. You can be sensitive to natural beauty products just as you might be to commercial products. If you have a known food allergy, such as to tomatoes, chances are you will also be allergic to cosmetic products that contain tomatoes. Care should always be taken when using a new product or treatment. Always spot test it first: Apply a small amount of the new product to the skin on the inside of your arm and wait twenty-four hours. If there is no reaction, it is probably safe to proceed with the treatment. If you are extremely sensitive, it is always best to consult a dermatologist or physician before using any new product or treatment. Remember, you are the manufacturer of these cosmetic products and quality control becomes your responsibility. Always work with clean equipment and pure ingredients.

The following is a list of basic care and storage guidelines to ensure a long and healthy shelf life for your homemade cosmetic products:

1. Always store your products in clean jars and bottles.

2. Try to keep your fingers out of the container as much as possible. Always wash your hands before handling cosmetics. Remember, when you dip your fingers into the containers, foreign germs and materials can be introduced. Try to use cotton balls, cotton swabs, or a small spatula when possible, or pour your products onto clean hands.

3. Store your products in a cool, dark, dry place. Heat and light can sometimes alter the composition of your products.

4. If the products separate, don't worry—they can usually be saved. Simply stir the mixture thoroughly or reblend with a hand mixer or blender.

5. If something smells bad (a strong sour odor, for example), it probably is. Throw it out. Once a product has gone bad, there is no way to recover it. You are safer making a new batch.

Equipment and Ingredients

The following is a list of the tools you will need for making your own cosmetics and beauty treatments. Many are common kitchen items that you probably already own. You will not need all of the items listed — for example, a blender, electric mixer, or spoon can be used for stirring. Remember to always keep your equipment clean; you don't want to introduce any foreign ingredients into your cosmetic products.

Grater: For grating beeswax, soap, and vegetables.

Vegetable peeler: For peeling vegetables and grating beeswax and soap. I prefer to use a vegetable peeler for grating beeswax and cocoa butter since it is quicker and the peeler is easier to clean than a grater.

Citrus peeler and zester: For peeling citrus fruits and removing the zest, or colored part of the peel. This is not necessary but is a fun gadget to use. You can do just as well with a sharp paring knife.

Knives: For cutting and chopping.

Measuring cups and spoons: Essential for measuring ingredients correctly.

Glass ovenproof measuring cups with pouring spouts: I use these for everything. They can be put in a hot-water bath, the microwave, and the refrigerator. Glass will not react with any of your cosmetic ingredients and is easy to clean.

Stirring rod: I use a chopstick for a stirring rod. It isn't essential, but it makes stirring small amounts easy. It also makes me feel like more of a chemist.

Pans: Steel and enamel pans work best. Aluminum and iron sometimes react with ingredients, especially when making soap.

Old muffin or loaf pans: Used as molds when making soap.

Blender and/or food processor: Perfect for really mixing up creams and lotions. You can mix pretty well by hand, but a blender makes the task so much easier and faster. Make sure your blender is dishwasher-safe to cut down on cleaning time.

Hand mixer or electric whisk: Speeds up mixing of creams and lotions as does a blender, but because it is handheld you have a little more direct control.

Coffee grinder: For grinding peels and herbs. Make sure you clean it well after each use or your coffee may taste a bit funny!

Funnel: For bottling your products and filtering solutions.

Coffee filters, cheesecloth, paper towels: Place in funnels for filtering solutions and mixtures.

Glass and ceramic bowls: For mixing, heating in the microwave, and storing products.

Eyedropper: For adding scents and natural preservatives.

Strainer: For straining solutions and mixtures.

Stove top, hot plate, or electric skillet: You will need heat to melt ingredients in some of the recipes. If you do not have a stove available, you can use an electric skillet filled with one to two inches of water to create a water bath.

Microwave oven: Not entirely necessary, but really speeds up heating and melting times.

Assorted jars, bottles, bowls, and spray bottles: For storing and applying your cosmetics. These containers can be found in a variety of places: grocery stores, drugstores, department stores, and stores specializing in cooking equipment. Put your recycling creativity to use—before you throw out an old jar, bottle, or container, think of how it could be reused for your home cosmetics. Honey bears and mustard squeeze bottles are great for lotions, shampoos, and liquid soaps. Wine and liquor bottles are perfect for scented oils and bath mixtures. Even your old commercial cosmetic containers can be used to hold your new homemade versions.

BEAUTY SHOPPING

Shopping for ingredients can be as much fun and exciting as making your own cosmetics. Many of them you are probably already buying and using, such as vegetable oils, water, eggs, yogurt, avocados, salt, cornstarch, vinegar, baking soda, and mayonnaise. Some of the ingredients in this book may be new and unfamiliar to you, such as witch hazel, castile soap, cocoa butter, lanolin, rose water, and essential oils. But these ingredients are also easy to find. Many are already at your corner grocery or drugstore and you have been walking past them.

You may have to break out of your standard shopping routine and explore new stores. This is where your adventure begins. I love to wander down the aisles of a new grocery store, natural food store, or farmers' market. This is where I get much of my inspiration for new recipes or new twists on age-old favorites.

Don't be shy about talking to the people working in the store. Usually they are as interested in what you are buying as you are in what they are selling. I am often asked in liquor stores what I plan on doing with my vodka, rose water, and orange flower water! I also like to find out where *they* get their products, and what their other customers do with them.

Looking for some of the more exotic products called for in this book such as green French clay or dried kelp may be frustrating at times. Use the telephone to call merchants and save time and energy. You may even want to keep a small notebook of what stores in your town or neighborhood have which ingredients.

I shop for ingredients in four different types of stores: grocery stores, natural food stores, pharmacies, and specialty stores such as liquor stores or bee supply stores. Depending on where you live, many supermarket chains have superstores that also combine natural food stores, pharmacies, and liquor stores for one-stop shopping. A good natural food store is worth the effort to find. I especially love the bulk bins where you can purchase many products at bargain prices. You may need to bring your own containers, so check ahead with your store. The pharmacy or drugstore can always be counted on for basic cosmetic ingredients such as witch hazel, lanolin, and mineral oil. Your pharmacist can also provide you with a wealth of information if you have a question about the purpose of an ingredient.

You may also need to go to specific stores for some special items. I buy beeswax at bee supply shops (where they sell equipment used by beekeepers), stearic acid powder from chemical supply houses, and special exotic herbs from herb shops.

Where you find items may vary. Your grocery store may have a wide variety of natural herbs and oils, and rose water may be found at a local gift shop. Now that you are looking for certain ingredients you will be surprised at where you see them sold. I have purchased essential oils in vitamin shops and beeswax at local farmers' markets. I have seen coconut oil on the cosmetic shelf as well as in the cooking section of many stores. Keep your eyes open and have fun. You may even discover a new ingredient. I found some blue cornmeal at a farmers' market the other day and love using it instead of the usual yellow meal. The results are the same, but the new color is fresh and different.

Another source of information and ingredients is the World Wide Web or Internet. This computer-based network of products, people, and services has become a valuable and easy-to-use source of information and products. I have found my own computer use has increased exponentially! I used to log on every now and then just to check out what was new—now I cannot live without it. I even have my own website, which has become a valuable source of information for my readers and myself. I have found simply searching on an ingredient or product produces an amazing amount of information. If you do not have Internet access, many libraries across the country are online and can easily help you learn more about this electronic resource.

BASIC NATURAL BEAUTY INGREDIENTS

The following is a list of the main natural products used throughout this book. You are probably already using many of them in one form or another. Many of them, such as beer, mayonnaise, and yogurt, I use all by themselves; I could not do without them. If you require more information, there are a number of excellent books on cosmetic ingredients—check with your local library—and many manufacturers provide detailed information if you call or write to them.

Almond oil: A pale yellow oil expelled or pressed from the seed of the sweet almond tree, it is rich in natural emollients that have skin-softening qualities. I purchase almond oil at the grocery store; it is found in the cooking oil section.

Aloe vera: The leaves from the aloe vera plant contain a sap that is believed to promote healing and soothe the skin. This sap is 99½ percent water. Many grocery stores stock aloe vera gel, as do pharmacies.

Alum (aluminum sulfate): In cosmetics, alum can be found in many astringents and aftershaves. It acts as an antiseptic and helps stop bleeding. Add a pinch to your favorite astringent or toner recipe to give it extra tightening power. You can purchase cosmetic-grade alum at drugstores or pharmacies.

Apricot kernel oil (persic oil): A light oil obtained from the kernels or pits of apricots, it is a popular body oil as it does not leave an oily film on the skin. This oil is a bit more difficult to find; I buy mine at a local natural food store.

Aspirin (salicylic acid): Salicylic acid occurs naturally in many plant leaves. People used to cure their headaches by chewing wintergreen or sweet birch leaves. Aspirin can be used as a preservative, antiseptic, and anti-itch treatment. Care should be used, however, as aspirin can be absorbed through the skin.

Avocados: Avocados are rich in natural oil, protein, and vitamins A and B. They contain more protein than any other fruit. In Mexico, women use it as a moisturizer to protect their skin and hair from the hot and dry climate. A simple and nourishing facial mask is made by mashing an avocado and spreading it on your face for fifteen minutes, then rinsing with tepid water and patting dry.

Avocado oil: A pale green oil made from the dehydrated flesh of the avocado, avocado oil is popular in cooking because it contains no cholesterol and has a very high smoking point. It is excellent for moisturizing the skin and hair because it has very high vitamin A and E contents and absorbs ultraviolet radiation from the sun. This oil can be found in the cooking oil section at the grocery store.

Baking soda (sodium bicarbonate): Baking soda is a gentle, alkaline, white powder that neutralizes acids. When mixed with acids such as vinegar, carbon dioxide is produced. This common household product is used as a skin soother, tooth powder, and deodorizer. It can be purchased at any grocery store.

Beer: Beer makes an excellent hair rinse and setting lotion. The flatter the beer, the better. The sugar and protein in beer work to thicken the hair. Don't worry about smelling like a brewery—the odor leaves as soon as your hair dries.

Beeswax: Beeswax is the wax secreted from the underside of bees, which they use to make the walls of the honeycomb. No synthetic product having all its properties has been developed. It is a valued ingredient in the cosmetics industry, as it will not become rancid and has germ-killing properties. In beauty products it forms a protective barrier on the skin to guard against environmental irritants and lock in moisture. I buy my beeswax from a bee supply shop. Look in your local yellow pages under "beekeeping equipment." I have also seen beeswax in many health food stores.

Borax (sodium tetraborate): Borax is a natural chemical substance found on alkaline lakeshores such as in California's Death Valley. It is used as a water softener, preservative, and texturizer. Because it is a mild alkali it gently cleanses without drying the skin. Borax powder can be found in the detergent section of the grocery store.

Castile soap: Castile soap is a mild white soap made with olive oil. It is named after the Castile region in Spain where it was developed. Real castile soap must be at least 40 percent olive oil. It can be purchased at many grocery and natural food stores in both bar and liquid forms.

Castor oil: Castor oil is made from the seed of the castor oil plant. This pale, unscented oil is an excellent oil for the hair, nails, and lips. As one of the few oils soluble in alcohol it is a good fixative for perfumes and colognes. This oil is usually found in the health-care section of the grocery store or at the pharmacy.

Chlorophyll: Chlorophyll is to plants what hemoglobin is to blood; it is a vital part of healthy plant life. It is well known for its deodorant properties and helps promote healing. You will probably have to check with a local health food store to purchase liquid chlorophyll, or check the recipe on page 228 to make your own.

Cocoa butter: Cocoa butter is a creamy, fatty wax that is solid at room temperature. It is obtained from the seeds of the cocoa plant. Chocolate lovers will enjoy cocoa butter's mild chocolate scent. It is an excellent skin softener and can be used alone or mixed with other ingredients. Many pregnant women use it on their stomachs to avoid stretch marks. Cocoa butter can be found in any drugstore. (Look for products that contain 100 percent cocoa butter.) I like to buy it in a solid stick, which makes it easy to rub on the skin and lips.

Coconut oil: Coconut oil is a solid white oil at room temperature. Today it is bought mainly for cosmetic use rather than cooking because it is 92 percent saturated fat. It preserves the skin and hair by providing a protective layer that locks in natural moisture. You can use it as a conditioner for your hair, skin, and lips. I have found coconut oil in the cosmetic section of health food stores and in the cooking oil section of many grocery stores.

Cornstarch (corn flour): Cornstarch is a fine, white, starchy powder made from corn. It soothes the skin and is believed to possess healing properties. Many people use cornstarch in place of talcum powder. It also makes a good thickening agent for creams and lotions. I purchase it at the grocery store; it's in the baking section.

Epsom salts (magnesium sulfate): Epsom salts is a fine white crystal powder that can be purchased in any drugstore. Soaking in these salts is soothing to sore muscles because the salts are mildly astringent. Some people also take epsom salts for indigestion.

Essential oils: Essential oils are highly concentrated aromatic extracts of different plants (usually a single plant). They come in a wide variety of scents, ranging from common ones such as peppermint to the more exotic patchouli and sandalwood. They are more expensive than other scents but are worth it as the scents are pure and intense, and will last for a very long time. I purchase these fragrant oils at health food stores or aromatherapy shops.

Extracts and flavorings: Alcohol is mixed with a substance to produce an extract. It is then used to scent and flavor mixtures. Extracts come in a wide variety of flavors, from banana to peppermint. If you need a quick and inexpensive cologne, they are easy to use; my personal favorite is vanilla. A wide variety of extracts can be found in the spice section of the grocery store.

Flowers: I love everything about flowers. Some of my favorites to use in cosmetics are marigold (calendula), lavender, chamomile, rose, gardenia, and pansy. You can purchase flowers fresh or dried from organic growers (you do not want any pesticides used on the flowers), or grow your own. Flowers that have wilted or turned a bit brown are still usable in cosmetic products. Flowers have been used in cosmetics for ages, oftentimes for symbolic reasons (for instance, lavender is believed to bring good luck to women). A flower's physical properties are also important; marigold, for example, has very strong healing powers because of its antibacterial properties.

Glycerine: Glycerine is a clear, odorless, sticky liquid produced during soap making. It attracts moisture and keeps products from drying out. If you read cosmetics labels you will notice it listed as an ingredient in many products. A classic hand-softening formula is glycerine and rose water. I purchase glycerine at the grocery store in the health-care section; pharmacies often carry it also.

Grape seed oil: This light, colorless, and unscented oil is expressed from grape seeds, and is a popular massage oil and cosmetic oil because it is so mild and hypoallergenic. It is also used as a hair conditioner and as a styling oil, which is believed to enhance hair growth. Grape seed oil is available at the grocery store in the cooking oil aisle.

Green tea: This tea has become a popular cosmetic ingredient because it is a strong antioxidant that many believe has antiaging benefits. As a facial rinse green tea tightens the pores and calms the skin. It is also added to creams and lotions to refresh and soothe the skin. There are many varieties of green teas depending on what part of the plant is used. The highest-quality tea is called *Gyokuro* and is made from the earliest tender leaves. Green tea is sold at many grocery stores; for more varieties you may want to shop at an Asian market.

Henna leaves: Ground henna leaves are a well-known ancient beauty treatment for the hair and nails. The henna plant or shrub grows in North Africa and the Near East. Henna contains a resinous substance that, when mixed with water, will coat your hair, skin, and nails. It can be used to dye the hair, give it extra body and shine, and strengthen the nails. Make sure the henna you purchase is made from 100 percent henna leaves. I purchase mine at the drugstore.

Herbal teas: Herbal teas are an excellent source of herbs such as chamomile flowers or a mixture of herbs. Make sure they contain pure herbal ingredients. Tea bags are also ideal for making scented waters and oils, as you do not have to strain out the solids. Herbal teas can be used in the bath, as skin fresheners and hair rinses, and in creams and lotions. Many grocery stores have a wide variety of natural herbal teas.

Honey: Honey is made by bees from the nectar of flowering plants and trees and contains many vital vitamins and minerals. It has a very high potassium content, which makes it almost impossible for bacteria to survive in it. Honey is one of the best-known humectants (materials that hold moisture). My favorite way to use honey is in the bath: a tablespoon or two makes your skin feel silk! Honey is available in grocery and natural food stores. There are many different varieties, such as clover or sage, based on what blossoms the bees find near their hive.

Jojoba bean oil: The jojoba plant is found in southern Arizona, southern California, and northern Mexico. On the jojoba shrub grows a pod that contains one to three seeds, 48 to 51 percent of which is oil. Jojoba bean oil has become very popular recently because it is very similar to our bodies' own natural oils. Native Americans and Mexicans have used jojoba beans for centuries. Many health food or natural food stores carry this oil.

Lanolin: Lanolin is found in the oil glands of sheep and is more like a wax than an oil or fat. It absorbs and holds water to the skin. There is no known scientific proof that lanolin penetrates skin better than oil, though many believe this to be so. I purchase lanolin at the drugstore.

Lemons (and all citrus fruits): The lemon is a very versatile fruit. It is commonly used in cosmetics because of its citric acid content. Citric acid kills bacteria on the skin. The fresh citrus scent is very popular and is a known energizer. The whole fruit is useful, from the peel to the acidic juice. I like to use lemons on a summer day to bring out the natural highlights in my hair. Lemon juice mixed with water also makes a super hair rinse for removing built-up gels and oils.

Macadamia nut oil: This is a relatively new cooking oil from Hawaii that is perfect for skin care use because it is so light and easily absorbed by the skin. I like to use it in place of other light oils such as sesame or almond in cream and lotion recipes. It can also be used alone as an after-bath oil. I purchase it at the grocery store, but it may also be found in gourmet cooking shops.

Mayonnaise: Mayonnaise is made from oil, eggs, and vinegar or lemon juice. The oil and eggs are moisturizing and nourishing to the skin, and the vinegar or lemon juice helps restore the skin's natural acid level. It is a complete treatment and can be used as a moisturizer for the skin or as a conditioner for the hair before the final rinse. Mayonnaise is found in any grocery store and is also simple to make at home (see recipe for Beauty Mayo on page 94).

Mineral oil: Mineral oil is widely used in cosmetics because it will not spoil over time, as do many other oils. It is a mixture of refined liquid hydrocarbons derived from petroleum. If you were to read the label on baby oils, you'd find that it is the main ingredient. Petroleum jelly is the solid form of this oil; it stays on top of the skin, providing a shiny protective surface. I purchase it at the grocery store in the health-care section.

Oatmeal: Oatmeal is a popular breakfast cereal rich in protein, potassium, iron, phosphates, magnesium, and silicon. It has gentle cleaning properties and can be used in place of soap. Oatmeal is nontoxic and soothing to the skin, so it's especially good for sensitive skin. It is found in the cereal section at the grocery store. "Regular" oatmeal (not quick-cooking) works best when making cosmetic products.

Olive oil: Olive oil was probably the first oil used in cosmetics. It is obtained from fresh, ripe olives and ranges in color from a pale yellow to a dark green. My brother likes to use olive oil mixed with vitamin E oil on his skin for an intensive skin treatment. It is found in the cooking oil section of many grocery stores.

Orange flower water (neroli): Orange flower water is a fragrant water made from the orange blossom of the bitter orange tree. It is also an excellent astringent and cleanser. The oil from this orange flower is called neroli, and its scent is believed to reduce stress and induce sleep. I find this water at the liquor store in the mixer section, or in specialty or health food stores.

Orrisroot powder: The root of the white iris (*Iris Florentina*) is used as a fixative in perfumes and powders. The dried root has a light violet scent, and its use dates back to Roman times. Many natural food stores carry this powder in their bulk bins. It is also very popular with those who make their own potpourris, so you may find it in craft or herb shops.

Rose water: Rose water is a fragrant water made from distilling fresh rose petals with water. Rose petals are astringent and cleansing. In London, rose water is added to champagne for a fragrant and special drink. I find rose water at the liquor store in the mixer section, but I have also seen it in the health-care section of many natural food stores.

Salt (sodium chloride): Salt can be found in any kitchen cupboard and is used as an astringent and antiseptic in cosmetics. It can also be used for removing dead skin from the body and scalp. I would not suggest using salt on your face or on irritated skin, as it can be very drying.

Sesame oil: Sesame oil is a pale yellow oil made from sesame seeds; it has a mild sesame scent. It has sunscreening properties, one of the highest for natural oils (only mink oil is higher). This oil can be found in the cooking oil section at the grocery store.

Soap: Soap is the oldest of all cleaning products. It is made with water, lye, and fat or oils in a chemical process called saponification. Shampoo and liquid soaps are diluted forms of soap mixed with water, glycerine, and other ingredients for the desired texture and results. Soap can be purchased everywhere, from grocery stores to fancy gift shops. It is usually inexpensive, and a good bar of soap will last for months. The soap industry is highly competitive; many manufacturers do not print the ingredients on the soap label. They do, however, print their name and address and many have toll-free numbers; you can call or write with any questions regarding the ingredients and use of their products.

Stearic acid: Stearic acid is a white, waxy powder obtained from animal fats and oils. When melted, it becomes a clear liquid. Stearic acid gives stiffness to creams and keeps the oils and water combined, much like beeswax does, but may be harder to find. I would look in the yellow pages under "chemical supply companies." Some candle-making shops also carry stearic acid.

Sunflower seeds: Sunflower seeds are rich in natural oil and vitamin E, which makes them perfect ingredients for skin scrubs, cleansers, and creams. If you grow your own seeds, the sunflower petals are also used in highlighting hair rinses and facial toners. These popular seeds and sunflower oil can be found at any grocery store.

Tea tree oil: Tea trees are an indigenous species of tree to New South Wales, Australia. They are fast growing, and the oil found within their leaves has powerful antibacterial and antiviral qualities. The tea tree has been used as a medicine plant for thousands of years by Australian Aborigines. Today nearly every Australian household has a small bottle in its medicine cabinet to help heal small cuts, scrapes, and bruises. You can find tea tree oil at your local natural food store and in some pharmacies.

Tincture of benzoin: A tincture is a solution that is about 50 percent alcohol. Benzoin is a gum resin secreted from the bark of the styrax benzoin tree, which grows in Thailand, Cambodia, and Sumatra. It is used as a preservative and antiseptic in cosmetics. I buy this at the drugstore or in the health-care section of the grocery store.

Vinegar (acetic acid): When fruit juice ferments, it turns into vinegar. Vinegars are known for their high acid content and sharp odors. In cosmetics, vinegar is used to remove alkaline residues from the skin and hair. You should never apply straight vinegar to your body; instead, dilute the vinegar with pure water (one part vinegar to eight parts water). Vinegar can be purchased at the grocery store.

Vitamin A: Vitamin A is found in fruits and vegetables, and can easily be absorbed through the skin (be careful, as too much can be damaging). It is believed to have skin-healing properties similar to those of vitamin E. Look for this and other vitamins at the drugstore or health-care section of many grocery stores.

Vitamin C (ascorbic acid): Vitamin C is used as a preservative and antioxidant in many cosmetics. It is also necessary in our diet for healthy teeth, bones, and blood. It can be found in many fruits and vegetables; most commonly in citrus fruits and broccoli. I buy mine in tablet form at the grocery store in the health-care section.

Vitamin E (tocopherol): Vitamin E is found in many vegetable oils. It is believed to protect body fat and tissues from breakdown and to slow down the aging process. It also helps normal red blood cells, muscles, and other body tissues to grow and remain healthy. Vitamin E oil can be used alone as a moisturizer; it is very thick and sticky and is best on small areas such as under your eyes. It can be purchased in capsule or oil form from a pharmacy.

Vodka (alcohol): Vodka is generally made from potatoes, but many cheaper vodkas are made from grains. The Russian name for vodka is *Zhizennia voda,* which means "water of life." Vodka is a good pure alcohol for making cosmetics; it's usually used as a solvent. Vodka made in the United States is ethyl alcohol (ethanol) and water. The percentage of ethanol is one half the proof; for example, a 90 proof vodka is 45 percent ethanol. I like to use natural alcohols, such as vodka, gin, and rum, in my products, as isopropyl (rubbing) alcohol vapors can make some people dizzy and sick to their stomachs. Vodka can be found in liquor stores, or, in some states, in the liquor section of grocery stores.

Water: Water is the major component of all living things and the ingredient used most often in cosmetics. The best beauty treatment of all is to drink at least eight glasses of water a day! Remember to always use the purest filtered water when making cosmetics.

Wheat germ oil: Wheat germ oil is a thin, golden oil with a very strong, nutty scent. It has a high vitamin A and E content and is believed to have healing properties. Like apricot kernel oil, this oil is a bit harder to find; I purchase mine from a health food store.

Witch hazel: Hamamelis virginiana, or witch hazel, is a plant whose bark and leaves are made into a wonderful skin freshener, local anesthetic, and astringent. Add witch hazel to your favorite lotion for a cooling moisturizer in the summer. My grandmother soothes her tired eyes by soaking two cotton pads in

SUBSTITUTIONS

I am constantly asked about substituting ingredients. Oftentimes readers can't find a particular ingredient or they do not have access to one or two ingredients. Sometimes it is a matter of personal taste or a known sensitivity to a certain ingredient. Substituting and experimenting are what home beauty is all about and why it is so popular. You are able to create the product you want and need using the ingredients you have on hand. I thought it would be helpful in this revised edition to offer a list of the more common substitutions. Many ingredient substitutions are easy to figure out. Many light oils can be substituted in recipes, resulting in very little difference to the end product. For example, if you are out of almond oil, try sesame, sunflower, or canola. Fresh fruits can also be exchanged with one another, as can dairy products, herbs, and spices. Of course you will develop a totally new product using the same recipe, but this is part of the fun!

Here is my list of common substitutions. (This is not a comprehensive list but a guideline to get you started.)

Ingredient	Suggested Substitution
Borax	Baking soda
Fresh herbs	Dried herbs (use half the amount of fresh)
Glycerin	Honey or light corn syrup
Lanolin	Coconut oil or vegetable shortening
Mineral oil	Any light vegetable oil
Orrisroot powder	Cornstarch
Petroleum jelly	Coconut oil or vegetable shortening
Rice flour	Cornstarch
Stearic acid	Beeswax
Tincture of benzoin	Vitamin E oil
Vodka	Gin, rum, witch hazel

witch hazel and resting for ten minutes with these pads over her eyes. It can be found in any grocery or drugstore.

Yogurt: Plain yogurt has wonderful skin-softening qualities. It is high in protein, calcium, and vitamins. Yogurt is easily absorbed by the skin and makes a soothing cleanser. I always keep a tub of it in our refrigerator. Yogurt is made by fermenting milk with special bacteria. (If you are really ambitious, there are many books and devices that allow you to make your own at home.) It is found in any grocery store in the dairy section.

Zinc oxide: Zinc oxide is a creamy white powder commonly found in ointment form and used as a sunblock. It is also used as an astringent, antiseptic, and skin healer. Make sure you purchase the United States Pharmacopeia (U.S.P.) grade intended for cosmetic use. I buy it at the drugstore.

BEAUTY TOOLS FROM NATURE

The following is a list of natural beauty tools that have been given to us by Mother Nature herself. Alone or grouped together, these beauty tools make a wonderful addition to your bath.

Loofah (Luffa) sponge: The loofah sponge has been used for years to remove dead skin cells from the body. Many commercial products today contain bits of loofah chopped up into fine pieces. The loofah is not really a sponge but a gourd that you can grow in your own garden. (Loofah sponge seeds are available at most garden shops and anywhere seeds are sold.) The seeds are slow to germinate, so sow early or start your plants indoors and then transplant. It takes about seventy-five days to produce a loofah sponge from seed. The plants like to have a trellis to grow on for support, and the mature fruit can be up to eighteen inches long. It is time to harvest your loofah when the skin turns brown. Dry the gourds in the sun, then soak them in water until the outer skin disappears. You will now have plenty of skin scrubbers to last the year, and home-grown loofahs make nice gifts. If you don't want to grow your own, you can purchase loofahs at any grocery or drugstore in the skin care section—they come in a variety of shapes and sizes. Some people also use them as natural pot scrubbers in the kitchen. *Never use a loofah sponge on your face, as they can be too harsh.*

To keep your loofah clean, wash it with mild soap and allow it to dry after each use. It is a good idea to get a new loofah every two months, especially if you use it every day.

Pumice stone: Our feet can thank volcanoes for this natural beauty tool. I grew up in southern Oregon, where pumice stones are everywhere. It was always fun to amaze your friends by lifting a pumice "boulder," as these stones are much lighter than they look. Pumice stones are supercooled bits of volcanic lava used to remove dead skin and calluses from the feet, knees, elbows, and hands. They always work best when wet. Soap the pumice stone and rub it gently over your skin. You can also use pumice powder added to your favorite cream (see recipe on page 44 for Pumice Scrub for the Feet). These stones can be purchased at any drugstore or pharmacy.

Cotton: Cotton is a very popular and important natural fiber. During the autumn months, fluffy white cotton bolls can be seen covering cotton fields in many southern and southwestern states in the United States. Cotton starts as a lovely white flower that blooms only for a day. As the flower withers and falls from the plant, a cotton boll containing the fluffy cotton appears. The cotton fibers are called the burr. Cotton is excellent for applying and removing beauty products because it is naturally soft and absorbent. Cotton balls and pads can be purchased at the grocery store or drugstore.

Sea sponge: The sea sponge is an animal that lives at the bottom of the ocean. Sponges are one of the oldest animals; for centuries, people have used their skeletons for cleaning and bathing because they are soft and absorb a large amount of water. You can purchase sea sponges at many drugstores and natural food stores.

Avocado pits: Inside the avocado there is a very effective massage tool — the pit. I like to rub an avocado pit over my arms and legs for a good massage treatment. Some people believe this helps remove cellulite. I know that it feels good and improves circulation.

Sand: Sand is a loose accumulation of tiny pieces of rocks or minerals. Beach sand is usually made up of calcite, which comes from broken shells and coral. In Hawaii there are gorgeous black-sand beaches that are made up of crushed bits of black lava. My feet never look or feel better than when I am at the beach, from all my walking in the sand and applying lots of lotion. Sand acts like a million tiny pumice stones to clear your feet of dead and rough skin.

WEIGHTS AND MEASURES

3 teaspoons = 1 tablespoon
4 tablespoons = ¼ cup
8 tablespoons = ½ cup
12 tablespoons = ¾ cup
16 tablespoons = 1 cup

1 cup = 8 ounces
1 cup = ½ pint
2 cups = 1 pint
4 cups = 1 quart
4 quarts = 1 gallon

juice of 1 lemon = about 3 tablespoons
juice of 1 orange = about ⅓ cup

METRIC EQUIVALENTS

1 ounce = 28.35 grams
1 gram = 0.035 ounce
1 quart = 0.946 liter
1 liter = 1.06 quarts

Cleansers and
Scrubs

*S*imple cleansers are used to keep the skin soft and clean by lifting off surface dirt and impurities. Soap is the classic cleanser but can sometimes be too harsh or drying for some skin types. There are many cleansing products that can be used as alternatives to soap. Oatmeal, for example, makes a mild cleanser. I like to use plain yogurt to clean my skin and keep it soft.

Cleansing scrubs are an important part of the natural beauty regime. They exfoliate or remove dead skin cells, which improves the texture of the skin and allows it to retain more moisture. This, in turn, enhances the efficiency of moisturizing lotions and creams. Depending on your skin type, cleansing scrubs should be used two to three times a week to keep the skin clean and healthy. Scrubs are not limited to the face; they can be used all over the body to keep skin soft and glowing. Don't forget classic rough skin areas such as knees, heels, and elbows. When making scrubs to use on your face, grind the ingredients as finely as possible. Treat your skin with care and gently scrub in a circular motion. Rinse the skin thoroughly and always pat, never rub, your skin dry.

The products contained in this chapter require the general care and storage guidelines found on page 8.

NATURAL SOAP ALTERNATIVES

If your skin is taut and dry, you may be using too strong a soap or cleanser for your skin type. Many of us grew up using "soap and water" to cleanse our face and body and have not explored non-soap alternatives. There are several natural ingredients that can be used in place of the traditional bath soap to get your skin clean and glowing and with beautiful results. Here are a few of my favorites:

Oatmeal: This common breakfast grain is probably the most popular non-soap cleanser around. It is gentle and mild and can be used by all skin types, especially those with dry and sensitive skin. To use, simply grind whole oats in a food processor or blender until you have a fine powder. Mix this with a little water to form a paste and massage this mixture into your skin with a warm washcloth. You may also add ½ cup of ground oatmeal to a warm bath to treat and cleanse your whole body.

Sugar: Granulated sugar works well as a gentle skin cleanser and scrub. It is not at all dehydrating and is perfect for dry skin types. Mix one teaspoon with a bit of water to form a paste and massage into wet skin with a warm washcloth or your fingertips. Sugar is gentle enough for your face and whole body.

Honey: Used as a skin beautifier since Egyptian times, honey is an excellent skin cleanser. It can be used alone or mixed together with a bit of lemon juice for oily skin types and milk for dry skin types. Simply massage into wet skin as you would any liquid soap or cleanser and rinse well.

Milk: For clean healthy skin, milk is an instant beautifier both inside and out. It is rich in protein, natural fat, and lactic acid, all of which help clean and detoxify your complexion, leaving it soft and smooth. Make sure you rinse your skin well after cleansing, as you do not want to smell like spoiled milk. Other dairy products such as sour cream and plain yogurt also work well as natural cleansers.

Oatmeal Cleanser

Oatmeal is a well-known and popular breakfast cereal—and is also a wonderful skin cleanser. It is especially well suited for people with sensitive skin because it is mild and soothing. Friends of mine who are unable to use soap because it is too harsh or drying like this recipe because it is easy to make and gently cleans their skin.

1 cup warm water
½ cup oatmeal
1 tablespoon glycerine or honey
1–2 drops tincture of benzoin
   (optional)

Place all of the ingredients in a blender or food processor. Blend on high speed until smooth and creamy. Place in an airtight container.

To use: Place a small amount in the palm of your hand and gently massage into your skin. Rinse well with tepid water and pat dry.

Yield: 8 ounces

Cleansing Milk

This is a common cleanser that is good for dry skin types. The yogurt and oil help to moisturize, and the lemon juice is a natural astringent that restores the skin's natural acid level.

½ cup plain yogurt
1 tablespoon sunflower or any
   light oil
1½ teaspoons fresh lemon juice

Mix together all ingredients. Store in the refrigerator.

To use: Pour a small amount in your hand and massage gently into your skin. Rinse well with tepid water and pat dry.

Yield: 5 ounces

Empress Josephine's Cleanser

¼ cup aloe vera gel
2 tablespoons fresh whole milk

Josephine de Beauharnais married Napoléon Bonaparte in France in 1796. She was known for her beautiful, clear complexion. It is rumored that she used this simple cleanser recipe every day to keep her skin clean and glowing. It is necessary to refrigerate this cleanser between uses because of the fresh milk. It should last for a few weeks.

Mix together the two ingredients. Store in the refrigerator.

To use: Pour a small amount in your hand and massage gently into your skin. Rinse well with tepid water and pat dry.

Yield: 3 ounces

All-Purpose Honey Cleanser

2 tablespoons liquid soap (Liquid castile soap works well.)
¼ cup honey
¼ cup rose water (Distilled water may also be used.)

Honey is one of my favorite ingredients because it is so versatile. I like to use this cleanser to wash my face and body, and I even use it to shampoo my hair. It does have a mild bleaching effect on your hair if used over a period of time, so keep this in mind if your hair is dark or color-treated.

Stir together all ingredients, being careful not to beat, as this will cause the soap to foam. Pour into a clean container; one with a pour spout or pump is nice.

To use: Pour a small amount in your palm and massage gently into your skin or hair. Rinse thoroughly with tepid water and pat dry.

Yield: 4 ounces

Olive Oil Cleansing Lotion

In ancient times, when clean water was scarce, olive oil was used to clean the body and protect the skin. It penetrates the skin very effectively to cleanse and moisturize. In the evening, after using this cleanser, I like to follow up with an application of more oil massaged into my skin.

Mix all ingredients together in a blender or by hand until smooth and creamy. Pour into a clean jar with a tight-fitting lid.

   To use: Put a small amount in the palm of your hand and massage into your skin. Rinse well with tepid water and pat dry.

Yield: 6 ounces

1 teaspoon liquid soap
2 tablespoons water
2 tablespoons glycerine or honey
½ cup olive oil

Arrowroot Cleansing Jelly

Arrowroot powder is similar to cornstarch in appearance and texture. It conditions the skin and allows it to retain more moisture. This recipe makes a clear jelly that could also be used to moisturize the skin. Cornstarch can be used in place of the arrowroot powder if you wish. The key to this recipe is to not boil the mixture or it will solidify after cooling and not spread as well into the skin.

Mix together all ingredients and stir until smooth. Heat in a double boiler or in a small pan placed in a water bath inside another pan. Heat until thick and clear; it will have the consistency of pudding. *Do not boil.*

   Let cool completely. If your cleansing jelly is too thick (a spoon will stand up in it), you may thin it by adding a little water, one tablespoon at a time, until you are happy with the consistency.

   Use in place of soap to clean your skin.

Yield: 4 ounces

2 tablespoons arrowroot powder (You may also use cornstarch.)
2 tablespoons glycerine or honey
½ cup water

Strawberry Cleanser

6 whole strawberries (cleaned; you
    don't have to remove the hulls)
2 tablespoons almond oil
3 tablespoons witch hazel

Strawberries make an excellent cleanser and moisturizer. They are rich in vitamins A and C—two vitamins necessary for healthy skin. Strawberries have a neutral pH like that of our skin, which makes them a good choice as a cleanser because they are so mild. If you cannot find fresh strawberries, frozen ones may be substituted. Make sure they do not have any added sugar and allow them to thaw before using.

Place all ingredients in a blender or food processor and blend until smooth. Pour into a clean jar and cover. You will want to keep this cleanser in the refrigerator because it contains real berries.

Use in place of soap to clean your skin.

Note: If you have oily skin, you may want to cut down on the amount of oil in this recipe.

Yield: 3 ounces

Grapefruit Cleanser

Peel from one grapefruit
½ cup olive oil
2 tablespoons grapefruit juice (Fresh
    is best, but bottled may be used.)
½ teaspoon borax powder

This cleanser is perfect for oily skin types because the grapefruit juice makes it mildly astringent. This is because like all citrus fruits, grapefruits contain citric acid. Any citrus fruit could be used in this recipe in place of grapefruit. Heat is used in this recipe to release all of the essential oils from the citrus peels.

Mix all of the ingredients together in a microwave-safe ceramic bowl. Heat for 2 minutes until very hot but not boiling by placing the bowl in a pan of boiling water or in the microwave on High.

Let the mixture cool completely. Pour the mixture through a strainer to remove all grapefruit peel. Store in an airtight container.

Use instead of soap to cleanse your skin.

Yield: 4 ounces

Country Fresh Dairy Cleanser

Milk has been used for centuries as a gentle cleanser and an alternative to soap. This is because of its lactic acid content, which helps deep cleanse your pores and kills any surface bacteria that may cause breakouts. This recipe uses whole milk to cleanse, condition, and stimulate your skin, leaving it fresh and glowing. If you have oily skin, you may want to use skim milk instead of whole milk.

½ cup water
¼ cup whole milk
2 tablespoons baking soda
1 egg white

Mix together all ingredients until well blended. Pour into a clean container.

To use: Pour small amount of cleansing milk onto a clean wet washcloth and gently massage into your face and neck. Rinse well with warm water and pat dry. Refrigerate any leftover cleanser.

Yield: 6 ounces

Gentle Eye Makeup Remover

Castor oil is excellent for removing eye makeup. I like to use this combination of castor, canola, and olive oils to remove my mascara in the evening. Even the most stubborn makeup glides off effortlessly with this light oil mixture. Castor oil is easily found at the grocery store in the health-care section.

1 tablespoon canola oil
1 tablespoon castor oil
1 tablespoon light olive oil

Mix together the three oils and pour into a clean container.

To use: Pour a small amount of oil onto a clean cotton pad and gently wipe over your upper and lower eyelashes and eyelids.

Yield: 1½ ounces

Almond Cleansing Scrub

1 tablespoon finely ground almonds
  or 1 tablespoon almond meal
1 tablespoon Almond Oil Lotion (see
  page 67) or your favorite cold
  cream (see pages 63–66)
1 teaspoon honey

*A*lmond seeds or nuts can be made into a cleansing scrub that gently removes dead skin cells from the face and is very soothing to the skin. It is important to grind the nuts into a fine powder, as large pieces could damage delicate skin (you can do this by hand or with a coffee grinder). You can purchase ground almond meal in some grocery stores if you do not wish to grind your own.

Mix all of the ingredients together. Store in a clean container.

   To use: Massage into face and neck; the mixture will seem a bit rough because of the ground almonds. Rinse well with tepid water and pat dry.

Note: I have found that almonds crush very easily if frozen first.

Yield: approximately 2 ounces

Favorite Cleansing Grains

2 tablespoons oatmeal
2 tablespoons cornmeal
2 teaspoons wheat germ

*W*henever I ask women what their favorite cleansing scrub is, I usually get three answers: oatmeal, cornmeal, or wheat germ. I have combined all three of these grains into one all-purpose mixture that you can use on your face and body. I like to keep a jar in my bathroom — I take a small amount and mix together with soap and water for extra cleansing power and to remove dead skin cells.

Mix all three ingredients together and store in an airtight container.

   To use: Combine a teaspoon or two of the mixture with equal parts water or cleanser to create a paste (you will need about ½ cup for your whole body). Massage this paste gently into your skin. Rinse well with tepid water and pat dry.

Yield: 2 ounces

Orange Peel Scrub

Whenever I use an orange or lemon in the kitchen I never discard the peel—I save it to use in my cosmetic products. Orange peel makes a highly effective facial and body scrub, since all of the essential oils of the orange are contained in the peel. Dried orange peel can be purchased in the spice section of your supermarket, or can easily be made in your kitchen. I like to use this scrub mixed with plain yogurt to clean my face. Other citrus peels also work well in this recipe.

Orange peels (You can make this recipe with one peel or several.)

Remove the orange-colored part of the peel; this can be done with a zester or a sharp paring knife. Dry the peels thoroughly; this can be done in four different ways:

1. Lay the peels on a rack to air-dry near a sunny window.

2. Place the peels in a microwave-safe ceramic bowl and microwave on Low until dry (about 5 to 6 minutes). Allow to cool completely.

3. Arrange the peels on a cookie sheet and place in a low-temperature oven (150 degrees) for several hours or overnight (remember to turn the oven off when you go to bed).

4. Use an electric food dehydrator and follow the manufacturer's recommendations for drying citrus peels.

Coarsely grind the dry peels in a blender or coffee

grinder until they're the consistency of coffee grounds or fine cornmeal. Place the ground peels in a clean bowl. Leave out to air-dry further if they are not completely dry after grinding.

Use the ground peels mixed in equal amounts with water or your favorite cleansing product. Other cleansing grains such as oatmeal and cornmeal can also be added to the orange peel for extra cleansing power.

Yield: each orange makes approximately 2 ounces

Avocado Stone Scrub

2–3 clean avocado pits (Make sure they are well rinsed of any avocado fruit.)

I used to grow all of the avocado pits or stones my family discarded. I would stick toothpicks in them and place them in jars of water. At one time I must have had fifty avocado plants (in various stages) growing in my bedroom. Then one day I read that these pits contained many of the same skin-softening and conditioning powers that the fruit and oil did and could help remove dead, flaky skin. I was thrilled—not only would I have more shelf space, but I had discovered a new beauty product! Now, instead of growing avocado trees I grind up the stones for a never-ending supply of Avocado Stone Scrub.

Place the clean avocado pits in a clean, sealable plastic bag. With a hammer or mallet crush the pits into small pieces (about the size of peas). Spread the crushed pits out on a clean plate or cookie sheet and allow to dry for a few days.

When dry, grind the pits into a fine scrub (the size of coffee grounds) using a food processor or coffee grinder. Again spread the scrubbing grains out on a plate or cookie sheet and allow to dry completely.

Store the scrub in a clean, airtight container. (I use resealable plastic bags. Make sure the scrub is completely dry before sealing the bag.)

You can add the ground avocado pits to your favorite cream, such as the Alligator Pear Lotion (see page 80), or liquid soap and massage into your skin to remove dead, flaky skin.

Yield: approximately 3–4 ounces

Apricot Kernel Scrub

Apricot kernel scrubs are very popular, and there are many commercial ones available today—but it is very easy and cost-effective to make your own. Apricots are an excellent source of vitamin A, which is essential for healthy skin. If you crack open an apricot pit, you will find a soft, ivory-colored nut or kernel. It is important that you discard the tough outer shell, as it is too sharp to use and could damage your skin. You can also use peach and nectarine pits in this recipe.

5–6 apricot pits

Wash and dry the apricot pits. Place the pits inside a clean plastic bag. Gently crack open the pits by hammering them on a hard surface. Inside the tough outer shell is an almond-shaped kernel. Carefully remove the outer shell and discard. Continue to pound the apricot kernels until you have a nice scrubbing powder the consistency of finely ground coffee.

Store the kernels in a clean container. It does not have to be airtight, as they will continue to dry.

Use the apricot kernel scrub alone or mixed with your favorite soap or cleansing cream.

Yield: approximately 2 ounces

Sublime Sunflower Scrub

½ cup raw sunflower seeds, shelled
Distilled water for mixing

Sunflowers growing in your garden guard it against pests and give you good luck — their seeds also make an excellent facial scrub. This treatment can be used to cleanse your skin, leaving your face incredibly soft and smooth. Sunflower seeds are rich in vitamin E oil. You may also use this recipe for an all-over, full-body treatment. Please note, you do not have to grow your own seeds to enjoy this recipe; they can easily be found at any grocery store.

In a food processor or coffee grinder, process the raw seeds until you have a fine powder that resembles coarse sugar. Pour this powder into a clean container with a tight-fitting lid.

To use: Mix 1 tablespoon of the ground sunflower seeds with a few teaspoons of water to create a smooth paste. You can do this in the palm of your hand or in a small ceramic bowl. Massage this mixture into your face and neck and rinse well with warm water first, followed by cool water. Pat your skin dry with a soft towel.

Yield: 4 ounces, enough for eight facial treatments or one full-body treatment

Sugar Scrub

Sugar makes a good abrasive skin scrub. It cleanses and stimulates the skin. Sugarbrasion is a popular treatment today at many health spas and beauty salons. I like to keep a sugar bowl next to my bathroom sink; when I travel I always keep a packet of sugar in my cosmetic bag.

1 teaspoon sugar
Soap and water
Juice of ½ lemon or 3 tablespoons
   Citrus Freshener (page 55)

While washing your face with soap, add a teaspoon of sugar to the lather and massage gently into your skin.

Rinse your skin with a mixture of equal parts lemon juice and water or the Citrus Freshener. Rinse with clear, cool water and pat dry.

Yield: 1 application

Oatmeal Elbow Cream

Nothing looks worse than rough, dry elbows. Stand in front of a mirror and really look at your elbows. If they do not look soft and smooth, then give them some attention! It is easy to overlook this part of the body, especially in the cold winter months when the majority of us wear long sleeves. This gentle cream is wonderful for removing dry skin from your elbows, knees, and feet.

2 tablespoons Basic Cold Cream (see
   page 63)
2 tablespoons oatmeal

Mix the cold cream and oatmeal together.

To use: Rub a small amount into your elbows (or knees and feet). Leave on for 15 minutes, and wash off with tepid water. Pat dry and massage more cold cream into your skin.

Note: For a super-easy elbow softener, cut a lemon in half and sit with an elbow in each half for 20 minutes, rinse well, and follow with a rich moisturizing cream.

Yield: 2 ounces

Pumice Scrub for the Feet

1 tablespoon ground pumice powder
2 tablespoons of your favorite cold
  cream recipe (or use Basic Cold
  Cream, page 63)

This is an excellent scrub for removing tough, dead skin from your feet. If you do not wish to take a hammer to your pumice stone, clean beach sand can be substituted for the ground pumice. Do not use this scrub on your face or body, as it could damage delicate skin.

To make ground pumice powder: Take an old pumice stone and place it in a heavy resealable storage bag. With a hammer, gently pound the stone until the pieces resemble coarsely ground pepper or beach sand. Mix the pumice powder and cold cream into a smooth paste.

To use: Massage the pumice scrub cream into your feet, giving special attention to your heels. Wash the scrub completely from your feet. I sometimes apply before taking a shower, but be careful, as your feet will be slippery. Afterward, apply more cold cream on your feet.

Store any leftover scrub in a clean jar with a tight-fitting lid.

Yield: 1 ounce

Astringents, Toners, and Skin Fresheners

*A*stringents, toners, and skin fresheners are important to healthy skin because they keep the surface clean and free of dirt, oils, and dead skin cells. The cleaner the surface of your skin, the more efficient it is at absorbing and retaining moisture. I like to use an astringent on my face after I wash it with soap and water to remove all traces of the residue from my skin. Toners and skin fresheners are also great to use throughout the day, especially if you have oily skin, so I keep a spritzer bottle of a water-based skin freshener in my purse. One of my favorite free skin fresheners is pure, cold water. Splash your face with cold water twenty times and count each splash. If you have very dry skin, you should limit the use of products with a high alcohol content and use those that contain more water.

The recipes in this chapter are extremely easy to prepare. They should be applied to the skin with clean cotton balls or pads; they can also be sprayed or splashed onto the skin.

Because many of these products contain alcohol, they have a long shelf life (the alcohol helps kill germs and bacteria). The products in this chapter require the general care and storage guidelines found on page 8.

Basic Astringent

¼ teaspoon borax powder
3 tablespoons distilled water
3 tablespoons rose water or orange
    flower water or distilled water
1 tablespoon vodka or witch hazel

This is an excellent astringent for your everyday needs. You can use it after washing your face with soap or cream to remove all traces of cleanser, or throughout the day to keep your skin fresh, especially after exercising. This recipe has a light floral scent; you may substitute distilled water for the rose water if you prefer an unscented product.

Dissolve the borax in the water, stirring well. Add the rose water and vodka. Stir well.

Bottle in a container with a lid so the alcohol will not evaporate. Apply to your skin using a clean cotton ball.

Yield: approximately 3½ ounces

Astringent for Sensitive Skin

4 tablespoons rose water
2 tablespoons orange flower water
2 tablespoons witch hazel

This astringent is good for dry or sensitive skin because it contains witch hazel, which is not as drying as pure alcohol. This is my personal favorite recipe and the one I use every day.

Mix all of the ingredients together. Bottle in an airtight container.

Apply to your skin using a clean cotton ball.

Yield: 4 ounces

Apple Juice Astringent

An apple a day will keep your skin glowing and clean. Apple juice contains pectin, which is soothing to the skin. This astringent will make your skin feel smoother and tighter, and it also has a nice mild apple scent. Pear juice works equally well in this recipe.

1/4 cup pure apple juice (no sugar added; fresh is best)
2 tablespoons vodka
2 tablespoons witch hazel } or 4 tablespoons witch hazel

Mix all of the ingredients together. Bottle in an airtight container.

Apply to your skin using a clean cotton ball.

Yield: 4 ounces

Strawberry Leaf Astringent

Strawberry leaves are a symbol of perfection and completion. The leaf of the strawberry plant contains four times the vitamin C of oranges. Next time you are cleaning strawberries for a meal, save the leaves for your own beauty treatments —you can dry the leaves yourself by putting them in the sun or by using a food dehydrator. This astringent is especially good for oily skin because it is a bit more acidic and drying.

2 tablespoons dried strawberry leaves or 1/3 cup fresh leaves
1/4 cup apple cider vinegar
1/4 cup rose water

Place the strawberry leaves and vinegar in a ceramic bowl and let sit overnight.

In the morning, strain the mixture and discard the leaves. Add the rose water to the vinegar solution and stir. Bottle in an airtight container.

Apply to your skin using a clean cotton ball.

Yield: 4 ounces

Orange-Mint Toner

1 tablespoon dried mint leaves or
   3 tablespoons fresh mint leaves
2 cups boiling water
Peel from 1 orange (orange part
   only—use a zester or sharp knife)
1 tablespoon vodka or witch hazel

When I was a young girl, I used to stick peppermint sticks in fresh oranges and drink the cool, sweet, tart juice. This recipe reminds me of that childhood treat—the mint and orange combine to give the skin a fresh, cool feeling. Mint leaves are rich in iron and the menthol helps tighten skin pores. This toner will whisk away surface dirt, oil, and dead skin cells from your skin.

Place mint leaves in a heat-resistant bowl and pour 1 cup of the boiling water over them. Let sit until completely cooled. Place the orange peel in another heat-resistant bowl and pour the remaining boiling water over it. Let sit until completely cooled.

Combine the mint water, orange water, and alcohol in the following proportions:

> ¼ cup mint water
> ¼ cup orange water
> 1 tablespoon vodka or witch hazel

Bottle in an airtight container, and apply to your skin using a clean cotton ball.

Note: Any remaining mint or orange water can be enjoyed in a spray bottle as a freshener for skin and hair. Or try using this water in one of your favorite face cream recipes.

Yield: approximately 4½ ounces

Honey Toner

1 tablespoon honey
1 teaspoon fresh lemon juice
1 tablespoon rose water
2 tablespoons vodka or witch hazel

As a cosmetic product, honey is very precious. It is a skin softener and a reputable healer. Put a small amount of pure honey directly on a skin blemish as a quick and easy remedy to help it disappear. It also makes a good skin toner, as it is a natural humectant that helps the skin retain moisture.

Mix all of the ingredients together. Pour into a clean bottle with a lid.

Apply to your face using a clean cotton ball.

Note: The toner may feel slightly sticky at first. This stickiness tends to disappear the longer the solution sits (this takes about 5 days). You may want to rinse your face with cool water the first week of use.

Yield: approximately 2 ounces

Cooling Cucumber Toner

¼ cup fresh cucumber juice (made by chopping up one cucumber, peel and all, and liquefying in the blender, then straining off the clear green juice)
2 tablespoons witch hazel
2 tablespoons distilled water
1 tablespoon vodka (optional)

Cucumber juice is a natural astringent. For sore or tired eyes you can soak two cotton pads in this toner and place over your eyelids while you rest. It also makes a mild tonic for sunburned skin. Cucumber juice is very delicate and spoils easily, so I suggest storing this toner in the refrigerator.

Mix all of the ingredients together. Pour into a clean bottle with a lid.

Apply to your face using a clean cotton ball.

Note: You may also want to filter this toner if you see solids (cucumber peel sediment) settling in the bottom of your bottle.

Yield: 4½ ounces

Mint-Vinegar Toner

1 tablespoon dried mint leaves or
   3 tablespoons fresh mint leaves
2 tablespoons apple cider vinegar
1 cup distilled water

Vinegar is a common household product that is used in many cosmetic products. It can be used in the bath, as a hair rinse, and as a skin toner. It helps restore acidity to the skin, keeping it toned and resistant to infection. All skin types benefit from using vinegar—it helps to control blackheads in oily skin and cures flakiness in very dry skin. Always remember to dilute vinegar with water when using it on the skin and hair (a good rule of thumb is eight times as much water as vinegar). I like to use apple cider vinegar in this recipe but white vinegar also works well.

Mix all of the ingredients together. Stir thoroughly and allow to sit for 3 days.

Strain or filter out all of the mint leaves. Pour the toner into a clean bottle with a lid, and apply to face with a clean cotton ball.

Yield: 8 ounces

Fennel Seed and Honey Toner

2 tablespoons vodka
1 tablespoon fennel seeds
1½ teaspoons honey
2 tablespoons distilled water
   (optional)

At my local library there is a book on western folk medicine, which states that the combination of fennel seeds and honey is a cure for wrinkles. I created this recipe based on this concept, and my skin feels smoother and tighter every time I use it. I also love the mild licorice scent the fennel seeds provide.

Combine the vodka, fennel seeds, and honey. Stir well and allow to sit for 3 days.

Filter the mixture into a clean container by pouring it through a funnel lined with a coffee filter. You may now use the toner full strength (apply to your skin with clean cotton balls), or add the distilled water to dilute the solution.

Yield: 1–2 ounces

Green Tea Skin Toner

Green tea was brought to Japan by monks returning from their studies at the great Zen monasteries of twelfth-century China. At that time green tea functioned as an aid to meditation and health. Today, it is one of the most widely used nonalcoholic beverages in the world. It is also an excellent skin toner because it contains antioxidants such as vitamins C and E, which help to strengthen your skin's natural defenses. This toner works especially well as an anti-irritant and can be used to soothe aggravated skin or sunburn.

½ cup pure spring water or distilled water
2 teaspoons green tea leaves

Bring the water to a boil. Place the tea leaves in a clean glass or ceramic bowl. Pour the boiling water over the leaves and allow them to steep for 2 to 3 minutes. Strain the tea leaves and allow the liquid to cool.

To use: Apply to the face with cotton or gauze. Do not rinse off.

Yield: 4 ounces

Vitamin C Toner

1 cup witch hazel
1 teaspoon fresh lemon juice
Yellow peel or zest from one fresh
  lemon
3 fresh or dried rose hips, slightly
  crushed

Vitamin C or ascorbic acid has become a popular cosmetic ingredient, and you will see several commercial products featuring this beauty vitamin. It is used as a natural preservative and antioxidant. In this recipe vitamin C is used to boost your complexion and fight the signs of stress by increasing your skin's circulation, leaving it radiant and refreshed. Fresh lemons and rose hips are both rich sources of vitamin C and naturally cleansing.

Combine the witch hazel and lemon juice. Place the fresh lemon peel and rose hips inside a clean container and pour the witch hazel mixture over them. Let this toner sit for a few days and then strain if you would like or leave the peel and hips inside your bottle for a decorative touch.

To use: Apply to clean skin with a cotton ball or spritz your skin with a fine mist spray bottle.

Yield: 8 ounces

Citrus Freshener

This is a light skin freshener to use throughout the day when your skin and hair could use a pick-me-up! I especially like to use this freshener when traveling by plane. I keep a small spritzer bottle in my purse to rehydrate my skin and hair. The clean citrus scent also gives me a boost.

2 cups boiling water
1 vitamin C tablet (a preservative)
Yellow peel (zest) from 2 lemons
   (Use a sharp knife or zester.)

Dissolve the vitamin C tablet in the boiling water. Place the lemon peel in a ceramic or glass bowl and pour the water–vitamin C mixture over it. Let sit for several hours or even overnight.

   Remove the peel with a slotted spoon, or pour the water through a funnel lined with a coffee filter to remove any solids from the liquid. Pour this water into a clean spritzer bottle and enjoy!

Note: This recipe works equally well with any citrus peel—tangerine, grapefruit, orange, or a combination.

Yield: 16 ounces

Chamomile Skin Freshener

In France, chamomile flowers are popular and are used in many products because the blossoms soothe inflamed skin and help stop dehydration. I use chamomile tea bags to make chamomile water, and I don't even have to use a strainer. Dried chamomile flowers work equally well in this recipe and can be purchased in bulk at many natural food stores. Substitute one tablespoon chamomile flowers for each tea bag.

3 chamomile tea bags (Use tea bags
   made with 100 percent chamomile
   flowers.)
2 cups boiling water
1–2 drops tincture of benzoin
   (optional)

Pour the boiling water over the tea bags in a ceramic heat-resistant bowl. Allow the tea bags to steep for several hours, until the mixture has cooled completely. Add the tincture of benzoin and stir thoroughly.

Bottle the chamomile water and enjoy; you may apply using a clean cotton ball, or use a spray bottle and spray your skin and hair.

Yield: 16 ounces

Gin Skin Tonic

1 tablespoon gin
3 tablespoons distilled water
2 tablespoons witch hazel
1 tablespoon orange flower water

At my parents' home in southern Oregon there are several large juniper trees; I used to spend hours climbing in and around them. Their blue-gray berries are perfect for making refreshing cosmetic products. Gin is a natural alcohol made from mashed grains and these berries. It has a distinctive sweet, clean scent. I love to use this skin tonic in the morning—the scent reminds me of my family home and those beautiful trees.

Mix all of the ingredients together. Pour into a clean bottle with a lid.

Apply to your face using a clean cotton ball.

Yield: approximately 3 ounces

Lavender Freshener

Lavender oil comes from fresh lavender flowers and is well known for its antiseptic or germ-killing properties. It takes an acre of lavender flowers to yield about twenty pounds of oil. Fresh flowers are placed in huge kettles over boiling water and the oil is distilled off. This recipe may be used on the face or splashed on all over the body after a shower or bath.

3 tablespoons distilled water
2 tablespoons witch hazel
2–3 drops lavender oil
½ teaspoon glycerine or honey

Mix all of the ingredients together. Pour into a clean bottle with a lid.

Apply to your face using a clean cotton ball.

Yield: 2 ounces

Beauty Water

My father-in-law once found at a garage sale an old book of formulas that was written in the early 1900s. In the book was an intriguing recipe for "beauty water." I have updated this old recipe and am quite pleased with the results. The original directions for use were as follows: "At night, before retiring, pour a teaspoonful in the palm of the hand and rub it over the face and neck, letting it dry. In the morning, an hour before the bath, repeat the operation, also letting the liquid dry. The regular use of this preparation for four weeks will give the skin an extraordinary beauty and freshness." You may follow these original directions or use the recipe below as a daily skin freshener. Because it contains egg white it should be kept in the refrigerator.

1 egg white
1 tablespoon glycerine or honey
1½ teaspoons vodka or witch hazel
2 drops lemon oil
2 drops lavender oil
2 drops oil of thyme

Mix together all ingredients. Place in a clean container and keep in the refrigerator.

Apply to your skin with a clean cotton ball.

Yield: 2 ounces

One-Minute Skin Type Test

Here is a simple test to find your skin type. For best results, do this procedure before cleansing your skin. Blot the oiliest areas of just one side of your face with a clean facial tissue; blot in several spots—your forehead, nose, and chin. Now examine your skin and the tissue:

Oily skin will show a considerable difference in gloss between the blotted side and the unblotted side. You will also see recognizable amounts of oil on the tissue. If you have oily skin you will be more prone to acne when you are younger and have fewer problems with dry skin as you age. You will want to choose lighter water-based cosmetic products.

Normal skin will show only a slight difference in gloss and very little oil on the tissue. As you age you will notice changes in oiliness and dryness and you may have to change your skin care routine. Normal skin types can use a variety of products both water- and oil-based.

Dry skin will display no difference and hardly any trace of oil on the tissue. Dry skin will require an increase in moisturizers and oils, as you get older. You will want to choose moisture-rich, oil-based cosmetic products and gentle alcohol-free cleansers.

Some people feel that they have combination skin because the center of their face is oily and their cheeks can be dry. The center part of your face is the oiliest for everyone and does not mean you have two skin types. Many skin-care experts disagree with the combination-type label. You are better off treating your skin as one type and using products designed for that skin type.

Creams and Lotions

The key to beautiful and healthy skin is keeping it clean and full of moisture. You will be delighted by how easy it is to create your own wonderful moisturizing products. Creams and lotions contain two basic ingredients: oil and water. Many creams use an emulsifier (a waxlike substance) to keep the oil and water from separating. Formulas without emulsifiers are just as effective; however, these have to be stirred or shaken before each use.

Dry skin is due not to the loss of skin oils but of water. Based on your skin type—oily, normal, or dry—you will want to adjust the amount of oil and water in the products you use. Dry skin types will want to use more oil-rich products, while oily skin types should use water-based products.

If you are uncertain what type of skin you have, there is an easy way to test it at home using a clean tissue. Follow the instructions for "One-Minute Skin Type Test" on page 58.

Some people feel they have combination skin, but you are better off treating your skin as one type or another. If in doubt, start with a good basic formula for all skin types and then adjust the recipe or product to meet your skin's needs. Skin type and character are constantly changing, and as you age your skin tends to get drier. I know that I can now use oil directly on my skin and it cries out for more; when I was a teenager I would never have done this. As you travel, your geographical location can affect your skin type; I use far less oil in a tropical climate than I do in an arid one. The change of seasons also affects your skin type; in summer I never seem to have a moisture-loss problem, since

I am constantly pouring lotions and oils onto my skin in the form of sunscreens.

The melting point of the oils you use in your creams will affect how greasy they feel on the skin. Oils with low melting points will feel quite greasy, whereas oils with high melting points will not feel greasy at all and will vanish into the skin.

Simple creams can sometimes be the best. My great-grandmother had beautiful skin at age ninety-eight, and she simply used a basic cold cream every day.

The products contained in this chapter require the general care and storage guidelines found on page 8. I have found that most creams and lotions in this chapter will last for eight months to a year. But I've usually used up the batch well before it could spoil. The recipes that contain real food ingredients will not last as long as those that are all oils—for example, products with eggs usually last only a few weeks. I do not double the recipes unless I am making them as gifts. This way you have a fresh product every four to six months.

Cold cream is the model for all creams and lotions; it's one of the oldest and best known of all beauty products. It is a mixture of oil, wax, water, and a mild alkali. The combination of oil and wax provides a cleansing action when it comes in contact with your skin; dirt and oil on the skin surface are loosened and can then be gently wiped off with a clean, soft tissue or cloth. Left on, it acts as an emollient to soften and smooth the skin and relieve dryness.

Dissolve the borax in the water in a glass measuring cup and set aside.

Mix together the oil and beeswax in another glass measuring cup. Place the glass cup in a pan of water (about 1 to 2 inches of water), making a water bath. Heat the oil-beeswax mixture in the water bath over medium heat until the beeswax is melted (8 to 10 minutes), stirring occasionally.

When the wax is melted, bring the borax-water mixture almost to boiling—I do this by putting the glass cup in the microwave on High for 1 minute. You may also heat it on the stove top in a water bath. Remove the oil-beeswax mixture from the water bath. Slowly add the borax-water mixture to it, stirring briskly. (You can also put the mixtures in the blender and whip.)

Pour the cream into a clean container with a lid. This mixture will last virtually forever—or at least until you have used it up. To use, massage a small amount into your skin and tissue off or rinse off with warm water.

Note: The mixture will become white and fluffy but will be a little runny until it has cooled completely. Once cooled, you will have a nice basic cold cream. Because you have not added any perfumes, it will remain

Basic Cold Cream

⅛ teaspoon borax powder
¼ cup distilled water
½ cup mineral oil or light cooking oil
2 tablespoons grated beeswax

unscented. If you choose to prepare a cold cream with a fragrance, just add a few drops of your favorite scent as the mixture is cooling.

Yield: 8 ounces

Original Greek Cold Cream

⅛ teaspoon borax powder
¼ cup distilled water
½ cup olive oil
2 tablespoons grated beeswax
1 teaspoon rose water

Cold cream was developed by the Greek physician Galen during the second century. It was called cold cream because as the water evaporated from the skin it gave a feeling of coolness. Mineral oil is used today in many products because of its long shelf life, but the original formula used pure olive oil, beeswax, and rose petal water. I prefer this recipe to the basic cold cream recipe because it contains olive oil, which seems to penetrate my skin better than mineral oil and does not feel as heavy.

Dissolve the borax in the water in a glass measuring cup and set aside.

Mix together the oil and beeswax in another glass measuring cup. Place the glass cup in a pan of water (about 1 to 2 inches of water), making a water bath. Heat the oil-beeswax mixture in the water bath over medium heat until the beeswax is melted (8 to 10 minutes), stirring occasionally.

When the wax is melted, bring the borax-water mixture almost to boiling—I do this by putting the glass cup in the microwave on High for 1 minute. You may also heat it on the stove top in a water bath. Remove the oil-beeswax mixture from the water bath. Slowly add the borax-water mixture to it, stirring briskly. (You can also put the mixtures in the blender and whip.) As the mixture cools, add the 1 teaspoon rose water and stir well.

Pour the cooled cream into a clean container with a lid. It will thicken as it cools. Massage a small amount into your skin and tissue off or rinse off with warm water.

Yield: 8 ounces

California Cold Cream

This cold cream combines two famous California products: avocados and lemons. It is the perfect antidote to dry, flaky skin.

For a lighter cream, take a portion of this cream (after it has cooled) and put it in the blender. On high speed, blend the cream, adding water one tablespoon at a time. If you end up with excess water do not worry—just strain it off your "fluffed up" cream. (This process works well with all of the cold creams in this chapter.)

Because this recipe contains real avocado and lemon, it will not have as long a shelf life as some of the other cold cream recipes. You may want to refrigerate this cream to keep it fresher longer. In the refrigerator it should last for up to four months.

⅛ teaspoon borax powder
¼ cup distilled water
1 teaspoon mashed avocado
1 teaspoon fresh lemon juice
1 teaspoon grated lemon zest
   (yellow part of the lemon peel)
½ cup avocado oil
2 tablespoons grated beeswax

Dissolve borax in water in a glass measuring cup and set aside.

Mix together the avocado, lemon juice, and lemon zest and set aside.

Mix together the oil and beeswax in another glass measuring cup. Place the glass cup in a pan of water (about 1 to 2 inches of water), making a water bath. Heat the oil-beeswax mixture in the water bath over medium heat until the beeswax is melted (8 to 10 minutes), stirring occasionally.

When the wax is melted, bring the borax-water mixture almost to boiling—I do this by putting the glass cup in the microwave on High for 1 minute. You may also heat it on the stove top in a water bath.

Remove the oil-beeswax mixture from the water bath. Slowly add the borax-water mixture to it, stirring briskly. Add the avocado-lemon mixture and continue stirring. (You can also put the whole mixture in the blender on high speed until well blended.)

Pour into a clean container with a lid. The cream will thicken as it cools. Massage a small amount into your skin and tissue off or rinse off with warm water.

Yield: 8 ounces

Cucumber Cold Cream

¼ teaspoon borax powder
1 tablespoon distilled water
¼ cup mineral oil (or any light oil)
1 tablespoon grated beeswax
1 tablespoon fresh cucumber juice
   (made by liquefying chopped
   cucumber in the blender and
   straining off all the solids; the
   result will be a clear green liquid)

The natural astringent powers of cucumber make this mild cold cream very effective. Like the Cooling Cucumber Toner on page 51, this cream contains fresh cucumber juice that can be very fragile and may spoil easily. To prolong the shelf life of this cream, I would suggest placing the container in the refrigerator.

Dissolve the borax in the water in a glass measuring cup and set aside.

Mix together the oil and beeswax in another glass measuring cup. Place the glass cup in a pan of water (about 1 to 2 inches of water), making a water bath. Heat the oil-beeswax mixture in the water bath over medium heat until the beeswax is melted (8 to 10 minutes), stirring occasionally.

When the wax is melted, bring the borax-water mixture almost to boiling—I do this by putting the glass cup in the microwave on High for 1 minute. You may also heat it on the stove top in a water bath.

Remove the oil-beeswax mixture from the water bath. Slowly add the borax-water mixture to it, stirring briskly. Add the cucumber juice to this mixture and stir thoroughly. You can whip the mixture in the blender if you wish.

Cool completely and pour into a clean container with a lid. The cream will thicken as it cools.

To use: Massage a small amount into your skin and tissue off or rinse off with warm water.

Yield: 8 ounces

Almond Oil Lotion

This is a light lotion with the clean scent of almonds. It makes an excellent hand and body lotion. I like to use it when gardening or working in water, as the oil and beeswax form a protective layer on my skin. This lotion is just the right consistency for my skin type, which is normal to dry.

⅛ teaspoon borax powder
¼ cup distilled water
½ cup almond oil
1 tablespoon grated beeswax
½ teaspoon almond extract
   (optional)

Dissolve the borax in the water in a glass measuring cup and set aside.

Mix together the oil and beeswax in another glass measuring cup. Place the glass cup in a pan of water (about 1 to 2 inches of water), making a water bath. Heat the oil-beeswax mixture in the water bath over medium heat until the beeswax is melted (8 to 10 minutes), stirring occasionally.

When the wax is melted, bring the borax-water mixture almost to boiling—I do this by putting the glass cup in the microwave on High for 1 minute. You may also heat it on the stove top in a water bath.

Remove the oil-beeswax mixture from the water bath. Slowly add the borax-water mixture to it, stirring briskly. (You can also put the mixture in the blender and whip.)

Allow the lotion to cool completely. Stir the almond extract into the cooled lotion if you would like more of an almond scent. The lotion will thicken as it cools.

Pour the lotion into a clean container with a lid.

To use: Massage a small amount into your skin.

Yield: 8 ounces

Australian Frangipani Lotion

2 tablespoons olive oil
2 tablespoons coconut oil
1 tablespoon light sesame oil
1 tablespoon almond oil
1 teaspoon grated beeswax
¼ teaspoon borax powder
¼ cup distilled water
1 tablespoon rose water
Several drops frangipani oil or
    frangipani fragrance (found in
    natural food stores)
3 tablespoons distilled water

The frangipani is one of the most beautiful trees in Australia, with a perfume that fills the air. It has clean, shiny, dark green leaves and clusters of creamy pastel flowers that seem to bloom year round. Frangipani trees are found in other countries under different names—plumeria, pagoda tree, or temple tree. This is a wonderful allover body lotion. I don't use perfume with this lotion, because I find the fragrance of the frangipani oil completely satisfying by itself.

Combine the oils and beeswax in a glass measuring cup. Place in a water bath and melt the oils and wax.

While the oils-wax mixture is melting, dissolve the borax in the ¼ cup distilled water. Add the rose water to the borax-water mixture.

When the oils-wax mixture has melted, heat the borax solution until just boiling (45 seconds in the microwave on High, or on the stove top in a water bath).

Remove the oils-wax mixture from the water bath and stir into it the borax solution. Allow the mixture to cool completely.

When cool, add several drops of frangipani oil. The more you add, the more fragrant your lotion will become. Remember not to add too much—you can always add more later.

Pour the complete mixture into the blender. On high, slowly add the 3 tablespoons distilled water, one at a time, until you have a light, white lotion.

Spoon into a clean jar or container with a lid. Massage this cream into your skin and enjoy.

Yield: approximately 8 ounces

Lecithin Moisturizer

Lecithin is often called "nature's emulsifier." (An emulsifier holds together two unmixable liquids, such as oil and water.) It is found in every cell of the body. Egg yolks contain a great deal of lecithin. Soy lecithin, which can be purchased in the drugstore, is made from soybeans. This is a light liquid moisturizer that you can use on both face and body.

1 tablespoon liquid lecithin
2 tablespoons light vegetable oil
1 teaspoon coconut oil
1 teaspoon mineral oil or light cooking oil
$1/8$ teaspoon borax powder
$1/2$ cup distilled water
1–2 drops of your favorite essential oil or fragrance, for scent (optional)

Mix together the lecithin, vegetable oil, coconut oil, and mineral oil.

In a separate container, dissolve the borax in the distilled water.

Gently heat the lecithin and oils until the coconut oil melts. (I put the mixture in the microwave for about 45 seconds on High. You can also heat the mixture in a water bath on the stove top.)

Heat the borax-water solution for 45 seconds on High in the microwave. If you are not using a microwave, you can heat the solution on the stove top in a water bath (fill a saucepan with about 1 to 2 inches of water).

Pour the heated solution into the lecithin and oils. Stir until well mixed. You can put the mixture in the blender and mix until smooth and creamy.

Add scent if you wish, cool completely, and pour into a clean container. Massage this cream into your skin.

Note: You can adjust the consistency by adding less or more water.

Yield: 6 ounces

Australian Lanolin Cream

2 tablespoons grated beeswax
2 tablespoons lanolin or coconut oil
½ cup almond oil or any light oil
2 tablespoons water
2 tablespoons witch hazel
⅛ teaspoon borax powder

Australia is well known for its wool production. One of the by-products of this industry is lanolin. Lanolin is the natural oil present in sheeps' wool. It is a popular ingredient in creams and lotions because it helps the skin stay soft and retain more moisture. Lanolin itself is 25 percent water. This is a recipe for a good general-purpose cream and works well on babies to prevent diaper rash. If you have a known sensitivity to wool products, you may want to substitute coconut oil for the lanolin in this recipe.

Combine the beeswax, lanolin, and almond oil in an ovenproof dish and heat until the wax and lanolin are melted. The best way to do this is in a water bath. Place the dish containing the wax, lanolin, and oil in a pan with 1 to 2 inches of water. Combine the water, witch hazel, and borax. When the wax, lanolin, and oil have melted, heat the water, witch hazel, and borax until just boiling. (You can do this in the microwave for 45 seconds on High or in the water bath on the stove top.) Slowly pour the water solution into the oil mixture and stir well. Pour into a clean container and cool completely.

To use: Massage into your skin.

Note: If you would like more of a lotion, simply add more water and witch hazel to the above recipe. I would start with double the amount of water and work from there.

Yield: 8 ounces

Basic Moisturizer

This is a recipe for a basic moisturizer. (Stearic acid is used to stiffen the cream and blend the oil and water.) It is a light cream with a velvety texture, perfect to use on your face during the day and under makeup. If you would rather not use mineral oil, any light vegetable oil may be substituted in this recipe.

¼ cup mineral oil or light vegetable oil
¼ cup stearic acid powder
½ teaspoon baking soda
2 tablespoons glycerine
1 cup distilled water

Combine the oil and stearic acid powder in a 16-ounce ovenproof glass measuring cup.

Combine the baking soda, glycerine, and distilled water in an 8-ounce ovenproof glass measuring cup.

Heat the oil and stearic acid in a water bath on the stove top until the mixture is a clear liquid and all of the powder has melted.

Heat the water solution until just boiling (about 2 minutes in the microwave on High or 5 minutes in a water bath on the stove top). Slowly add the water solution to the oil and stearic acid. You will see the mixture foam up as carbon dioxide is released.

Pour the entire mixture into a blender and blend on high for 2 minutes. The mixture will be a white, fluffy cream. Spoon the cream into a bowl and allow to cool completely.

When cool, stir again and spoon into a clean jar with a lid. Massage a small amount into your face and neck.

Yield: 12 ounces

Coconut Cloud Cream

2 tablespoons stearic acid powder
¼ cup coconut oil
½ teaspoon baking soda
½ cup distilled water
A few drops coconut fragrance
    (optional)

This is a light and fluffy cream that provides all the skin-nourishing qualities of coconut oil in a less oily form. I love to use this cream in the winter because the light coconut scent reminds me of summer and beach vacations. It is especially nice rubbed into warm skin after a bath or shower. Some women even put this cream in their hair for extra shine and conditioning. (I would suggest this only for people with very short hair.)

Melt the stearic acid and the oil together. You can do this in a water bath on the stove top.

Dissolve the baking soda in the distilled water and heat almost to boiling. (Put the solution in the microwave for about 1 minute on High, or heat in a water bath on the stove top.)

Stir the water solution slowly into the stearic acid–oil mixture. The mixture will foam up in volume (almost double); stir thoroughly.

Cool this mixture completely. When cool, add a few drops of coconut fragrance if you want a stronger scent (coconut oil already has a light coconut scent), and stir. Pour into an airtight jar and enjoy.

Note: If you cannot find stearic acid powder, you may substitute 1 tablespoon grated beeswax. Your lotion will not be as light and fluffy, but you will have a very nice skin cream.

Yield: 8 ounces

Corn Flour Lotion

This is a light, nongreasy lotion combining the old-fashioned formula of rose water and glycerine with corn flour. It is perfect for soothing dry, chapped hands. Corn flour is another common name for powdered cornstarch.

2 tablespoons glycerine
2 tablespoons corn flour (cornstarch)
½ cup distilled water
2 tablespoons rose water

Mix together all ingredients in an ovenproof glass bowl or pitcher. Heat until just boiling and thick, 1 to 2 minutes in the microwave on High (stirring every 30 seconds), or on the stove top in a water bath. The lotion will be clear and jellylike; stir thoroughly and cool completely.

When the lotion is cool, pour into a clean, airtight container. Massage into your hands, face, or body.

Note: If your lotion becomes too thick, don't worry— you can thin it by adding water, one tablespoon at a time, and stirring thoroughly.

Yield: 6 ounces

Body Butter

This is a rich, buttery cream that is a wonderful allover body cream. It contains four well-known skin-conditioning products: cocoa butter, coconut oil, sesame oil, and avocado oil. It is especially nice after a day in the sun or after a warm shower to lock in moisture. This is a heavy cream, and I would not suggest using it on your face.

¼ cup grated cocoa butter
1 tablespoon coconut oil
2 tablespoons sesame oil
1 tablespoon avocado oil
1 tablespoon grated beeswax

Combine all the ingredients in an ovenproof glass container. Place the container with the mixture in a pan with a 1-to-2-inch water bath. Melt the oils and wax gently.

Pour the melted mixture into a clean jar and allow to cool. Stir the cooled mixture.

Spread the butter on your body and massage into the skin.

Yield: 4 ounces

Grape Seed Oil Lotion

½ cup grape seed oil
1 tablespoon grated beeswax
¼ cup water
⅛ teaspoon borax powder

Grape seed oil is a light, nongreasy oil that is also hypoaller-genic. It is a popular natural beauty oil because it can be used by all skin types and is easily absorbed into the skin. I have seen grape seed oil sold in both the cooking oil sections and health care sections of grocery stores. It is basically the same oil, although the health care skin oil usually has a higher price.

Mix together the grape seed oil and beeswax and heat gently until the beeswax is melted. In a separate container mix together the water and borax powder and heat until very hot but do not boil. You may use the stove top or microwave to do this. Pour the oil mixture into a blender and start stirring slowly; add the water solution, and then mix on High until a thick lotion is formed. Pour the lotion into a cool container and allow it to cool completely.

To use: Massage into your skin as you would any rich moisturizer or cream.

Yield: 6 ounces

Papaya Cream

*I*n Australia, the papayas, or pawpaws, grow as large as melons and are delicious! Papaya is an excellent skin softener because it contains a great deal of papain, a natural enzyme. Unripe papayas have the highest content of papain; as the papaya ripens, the papain content decreases. I particularly like to use this rich cream on my rough hands, elbows, knees, and feet—nothing makes them feel softer. I would suggest storing this cream in glass or ceramic containers. (I have had it "eat" its way out of plastic containers because of the high enzyme content.) This cream contains actual fruit and it can spoil; store it in the refrigerator and it should last for about four months.

¼ cup almond oil
¼ cup stearic acid powder
1 tablespoon liquid lecithin
¼ cup fresh pureed papaya, can be unripe (I process the papaya in a food processor until it is a smooth cream.)
¼ cup distilled water
½ teaspoon baking soda
4 drops tincture of benzoin

Mix together the oil, stearic acid, and lecithin in an ovenproof glass container, and melt in a water bath on the stove top over medium heat. The mixture will become foamy and golden yellow as it melts.

Mix together the papaya, water, baking soda, and tincture of benzoin, and heat but do not boil (1 minute in the microwave on High or 5 minutes in a water bath on the stove top). Stir thoroughly.

Slowly add the papaya mixture to the oil mixture and stir thoroughly. The mixture will foam up in volume (almost double); keep stirring.

Cool completely and stir one more time. Place in an airtight container and use wherever you want softer, smoother skin!

Note: If you cannot find stearic acid powder, you may substitute 1 tablespoon grated beeswax.

Yield: 8 ounces

Refreshing Leg Gel

½ cup aloe vera gel
1½ teaspoons cornstarch
1 tablespoon witch hazel
3–4 drops peppermint oil

This is a light, nongreasy, invigorating gel that is perfect for tired legs and feet. It was a lifesaver on one summer trip to Singapore when I was eight months pregnant! For extra cooling action, place this gel in the refrigerator before using.

Combine the aloe vera, cornstarch, and witch hazel in a heat-resistant container. Warm the mixture until you have a clear, thick liquid about the consistency of honey. (You can do this in the microwave, stirring every 30 seconds for 1 to 2 minutes on High, or in a double boiler on the stove top.)

After the mixture has cooled, add the peppermint oil and stir thoroughly. Pour into an airtight container and enjoy.

Massage this lotion into your legs and feet for an instant, cooling pick-me-up.

Yield: approximately 4 ounces

Health Nut Lotion

¼ teaspoon borax powder
¼ cup distilled water
1 tablespoon wheat germ oil
1 tablespoon castor oil
1 tablespoon almond oil
1 teaspoon vitamin E oil
2 tablespoons grated beeswax

Wheat germ oil, castor oil, almond oil, and vitamin E all combine to make a rich lotion that heals and nourishes the skin. If you also enjoy a mild, nutty scent, this is the lotion to try. I use this lotion all over my body and as a night cream under my eyes.

Dissolve the borax in the water in a glass measuring cup and set aside.

Mix together the oils and beeswax in another glass measuring cup. Place the oils-wax mixture in a glass cup in a pan of water (about 1 to 2 inches of water), making a water bath. Heat the oil mixture in the water bath over medium heat until the beeswax is melted (8 to 10 minutes), stirring occasionally.

When the wax is melted, bring the borax-water mixture almost to boiling (put the glass cup with the mixture in the microwave on High for 1 minute, or heat it in a water bath on the stove top).

Remove the oil mixture from the water bath. Slowly add the borax-water to the oil mixture, stirring briskly. (You can also put the complete mixture in the blender and whip.)

Pour the lotion into a clean container with a lid, and cool completely. Use by massaging into your skin.

Yield: 4 ounces

Floral Aloe Vera Gel

I love to browse in the dried flower bin section at my local natural food store. Calendula flowers (marigolds) are a lovely shade of yellow-orange to red and have a sweet scent. Marigolds are a natural antiseptic. Lavender is also a natural skin healer that is good for burns and insect stings because it has a mildly sedative quality. This gel is an excellent skin soother, and the fresh floral scent is especially appealing and comforting.

½ cup aloe vera gel
1 tablespoon dried lavender flowers or 3 tablespoons fresh lavender flowers
1 tablespoon dried calendula (marigold) flowers or 3 tablespoons fresh calendula flowers

Mix together the aloe vera gel, lavender, and calendula in an ovenproof glass container. Heat the mixture gently. You can do this by placing the container in the microwave for 1 minute on High or in a water bath on the stove top.

Let the mixture sit and cool completely, then pour it into a clean container through a clean, fine strainer to remove all of the flower petals and solids.

Store in a cool, dry, dark location in a container with a tight-fitting lid. Apply to your skin.

Yield: 4 ounces

Cooling Aloe Lotion

½ cup aloe vera gel
1 tablespoon chamomile tea
1 tablespoon vitamin E oil
2–3 drops peppermint oil

The sap of the aloe vera plant is especially soothing to the skin because of its high water content (it is 99½ percent water). Chamomile and vitamin E also help condition the skin and prevent peeling if used on sunburned skin. This is a light lotion that I find very refreshing and cooling after a day in the sun.

Mix together the aloe vera gel and the chamomile tea. Heat gently, but do not boil, for 1 minute in the microwave on High or a few minutes in a water bath on the stove top. Let the mixture cool completely, and then strain off any solids and discard. Add the vitamin E oil and peppermint oil to the mixture and stir.

Pour into a clean jar with a tight-fitting lid. For a refreshing treatment, you can place the jar in the refrigerator to cool the lotion before using.

To use: Massage into clean skin. If your skin is sunburned, use gentle strokes.

Yield: 4 ounces

Witch Hazel Body Lotion

¼ cup sunflower oil (or any light oil)
1 tablespoon stearic acid powder
½ cup distilled water
½ teaspoon baking soda
2 tablespoons witch hazel

My mother once purchased a witch hazel body lotion that I loved to use—it was especially refreshing during the summer months. When it was all gone, we were disappointed to learn that the company had discontinued the lotion. Over the years I have experimented with different recipes, and this one comes closest to that original witch hazel body lotion.

Mix together the sunflower oil and the stearic acid powder. Gently heat the oil and stearic acid mixture in a glass container in a pan of water until the stearic acid has dissolved.

When the stearic acid has melted, mix together the water and baking soda. Heat the water solution gently until it is the same temperature as the oil mixture. (Put the water solution in the microwave for 1 minute on High, or use the stove top.)

Pour the water–baking soda mixture into a blender and blend on low. Slowly add the oil mixture in a thin, steady stream. You can also mix by hand, but I prefer using a blender, which is quicker and easier.

Allow the mixture to cool. When the lotion is cool, stir in the witch hazel. You can also add a scent at this time if you wish. Pour into a clean jar or lotion bottle with a tight-fitting lid.

Note: If you cannot find stearic acid powder, you may substitute ½ tablespoon grated beeswax.

Yield: 6 ounces

Allover Nighttime Lotion

This is a rich lotion packed with oils and vitamins. I like to massage it all over my body and face before going to bed at night. I wake up with really soft and smooth skin that looks and feels great. You can also use this lotion during the day as a moisturizer or eye cream.

Dissolve the baking soda in the water in a glass measuring cup and set aside.

Mix together the oils, lecithin, and beeswax in another glass measuring cup. Place the oil mixture in a glass cup in a pan of water (about 1 to 2 inches of water), making a water bath. Heat the oil mixture in the water bath over medium heat until the beeswax is melted (8 to 10 minutes), stirring occasionally.

¼ teaspoon baking soda
½ cup distilled water
1 tablespoon vitamin E oil
2 tablespoons olive oil
1 tablespoon avocado oil
½ teaspoon wheat germ oil
1 teaspoon liquid lecithin
1 tablespoon grated beeswax

When the wax is melted, bring the soda-water mixture almost to boiling—I put the glass cup with the mixture in the microwave on High for 1 minute. You can also use a water bath on the stove top.

Remove the oil mixture from the water bath. Slowly add the oil mixture to the water solution, stirring briskly. (You can also put the mixtures in the blender and whip.)

Pour the lotion into a clean container with a lid. The lotion will thicken as it cools.

Cool completely, then use this lotion all over your body.

Yield: 6 ounces

Alligator Pear Lotion

⅛ teaspoon borax powder
¼ cup distilled water
½ cup avocado oil
1 tablespoon grated beeswax

Alligator pear or butter pear are two nicknames given to avocados. My grandmother always used to call avocados "alligator pears," so it became my favorite nickname, too. Avocados are pear shaped with tough, scaly skin and are well known for their skin-softening and sunscreening properties. This is a rich body lotion with the benefits of avocado oil.

Dissolve the borax in the water in a glass measuring cup and set aside.

Mix together the oil and beeswax in another glass measuring cup. Place the cup in a pan of water (about 1 to 2 inches of water), making a water bath. Heat the oil-beeswax mixture in the water bath over medium heat until the beeswax is melted (8 to 10 minutes), stirring occasionally.

When the wax is melted, bring the borax solution almost to boiling (put the glass cup in the microwave on High for 1 minute, or use a water bath on the stove top).

Remove the oil-beeswax mixture from the water bath. Slowly add the borax solution to it, stirring briskly. (You can also put the mixtures in the blender and whip.)

Allow the lotion to cool completely. The consistency may seem a bit thin at first, but it will thicken as it cools. Pour the lotion into a clean container with a lid.

To use: Massage a small amount into your skin.

Yield: 8 ounces

Super Eye Cream

Vitamin E oil makes an excellent eye cream by itself, but I find it too thick and sticky (especially for day wear). This cream mixes vitamin E oil with cold cream to make an eye cream that is suitable for day or night use. Always apply eye cream with your ring finger; it is the weakest finger and will not pull the delicate skin around the eye.

1 teaspoon vitamin E oil (or you can break open 3 or 4 vitamin E capsules)
2 teaspoons Basic Cold Cream (see page 63)

Mix the vitamin E oil into the cold cream. Place in a clean container.

Apply around your eyes first thing in the morning and before going to bed at night.

Note: Although this is called an eye cream, I also use it on cuts and scars because of the healing vitamin E content.

Yield: approximately 1 ounce

Firming Neck Cream

2 tablespoons coconut oil
1 tablespoon macadamia nut oil
2 teaspoons apricot kernel oil
1 tablespoon cocoa butter
½ teaspoon vitamin E oil

Women take the time to care for their faces but often forget another very important part—the neck. This cream is rich in skin-conditioning oils perfect for the neck and throat. I like to massage it into my face and neck at night before going to bed, but if you have very dry skin, you can use it in the morning as well.

Mix together all ingredients in a clean, ovenproof container. Heat the mixture, gently stirring together all of the ingredients. You may place the container in the microwave for one minute on High or heat gently in a double boiler or water bath on the stove top.

Let the mixture cool completely. If you want a very solid cream, place it in the refrigerator to cool. This is especially helpful in warmer climates where the outside temperature may keep your cream from cooling completely.

Place the cream in a clean jar or container with a tight-fitting lid.

To use: Massage a small amount into your neck at night before going to bed.

Yield: 3 ounces

Tropical Eye Cream

2 tablespoons grated cocoa butter
3 tablespoons coconut oil

The sensitive skin under your eyes needs extra care and conditioning. Cocoa butter and coconut oil have been used for years to treat age lines around the eyes and mouth. They help to soften and protect delicate skin. This eye cream is rich, so a small amount is all that you need.

Mix the ingredients together in an ovenproof container. Heat gently in the microwave or in a water bath. Pour the melted mixture into a small clean container and allow it to cool completely.

To use: Apply nightly under your eyes to soothe and condition your skin.

Yield: 3 ounces

Yarrow Lotion

There is a story that Achilles used yarrow to heal his men's wounds after the Battle of Troy—yarrow, similar to chamomile as a skin soother, contains over 50 percent azulene, a well-known anti-inflammatory. It was also believed to be a "magic" herb by the early Saxons, who settled in England in A.D. 500. They wore amulets of yarrow to protect them from just about everything. I created this lotion to soothe a bad rash on my arms. It worked like a charm—my rash soon disappeared.

1 tablespoon dried yarrow flowers
　(Chamomile may also be used.)
1 cup boiling water
⅛ teaspoon borax powder
1 tablespoon jojoba oil
⅓ cup sunflower oil
1 teaspoon grated beeswax

Place the yarrow flowers in a heat-proof container. Pour the boiling water over them and allow to sit overnight or for at least 8 hours.

Measure ½ cup of the yarrow infusion and add the borax, stirring until well mixed. Set aside.

Mix together the oils and beeswax in a glass cup. Place the oils-beeswax mixture in a glass cup in a pan of water (about 1 to 2 inches of water), making a water bath. Heat over medium heat until the beeswax is melted (8 to 10 minutes), stirring occasionally.

When the wax is melted, bring the yarrow solution almost to boiling—I put the glass cup with the yarrow water–borax in the microwave on High for 1 minute. You can also use a water bath on the stove top.

Remove the oil-beeswax mixture from the water bath. Slowly add the yarrow water–borax to the mixture, stirring briskly. (You can also put the mixtures in the blender and whip.)

Allow the lotion to cool completely. The consistency may seem a bit thin, but it will thicken as it cools. The lotion will be pale yellow in color. Pour the lotion into a clean container with a lid.

To use: Massage a small amount into your skin.

Yield: 6 ounces

Mint Body Lotion

½ cup mint water (see Note on page 85)
⅛ teaspoon borax powder
½ cup sunflower oil
1 teaspoon coconut oil
1 teaspoon grated beeswax
3–4 drops peppermint oil (optional)

After a peppermint oil bath or shower this lotion is especially refreshing. Mint is a natural energizer, and if you are lucky enough to have fresh mint in your yard this is a great way to use it. If you don't, you can find it at any good grocery store. Peppermint or spearmint, or a combination of both, works well.

Mix together the mint water and the borax, stirring until well mixed. Set aside.

Mix together the sunflower oil, coconut oil, and beeswax in a glass measuring cup. Place the cup with the oils-beeswax mixture in a pan of water (about 1 to 2 inches of water), making a water bath. Heat over medium heat until the beeswax is melted (8 to 10 minutes), stirring occasionally.

When the wax is melted, bring the mint solution almost to boiling (put the glass cup with the mint water–borax in the microwave on High for 1 minute, or use a water bath on the stove top).

Remove the oils-beeswax mixture from the water bath. Slowly add mint water–borax to the mixture, stirring briskly. (You can also put the mixtures in the blender and whip.)

Allow the lotion to cool completely. The consistency may seem a bit thin, but it will thicken as it cools. The lotion will be pale green in color. You may add the peppermint oil now if you wish.

Pour the lotion into a clean container with a lid.

To use: Massage a small amount into your skin.

Note: Mint water is made by boiling fresh or dried mint leaves in water and then letting the mixture cool. Strain off the mint leaves. I use 1 cup fresh mint (¼ cup dried mint leaves) to 1 cup water.

Yield: 8 ounces

Mermaid Lotion

If mermaids had a beauty secret, it would be seaweed. It is very soothing to the skin and helps skin-cell renewal. Irish moss (Chondrus crispus) is a red seaweed found in the North Atlantic. It contains carrageenan, which acts as a stabilizer and emulsifier. I buy powdered Irish moss at natural food stores. Make sure you use Irish moss in this recipe, as not all seaweeds have the same characteristics. I have tried kelp powder, for example, and it does not gel.

1 tablespoon powdered Irish moss or
    any dried seaweed
1 cup distilled water
¼ cup aloe vera gel
2 tablespoons almond oil

Mix together the Irish moss and water and let sit for 20 minutes.

Pour the mixture into a small saucepan and boil for 20 minutes. Strain off the solids; you will have a clear jelly.

Measure ¼ cup of your seaweed jelly and mix with the aloe vera gel. Let the mixture cool completely.

Pour the seaweed mixture into the blender and blend on low speed; slowly add the almond oil in a thin stream until all is blended. You will now have a light, white lotion.

Pour into a clean container, and enjoy by massaging a small amount into your skin.

Yield: 4 ounces

Stretch Mark Cream

1/4 cup cocoa butter
1 tablespoon wheat germ oil
1 teaspoon light sesame seed oil
1 teaspoon apricot kernel oil
1 teaspoon vitamin E oil
2 teaspoons grated beeswax
1 teaspoon vanilla extract (optional)

I used this cream during and after my pregnancies to avoid stretch marks. Rub a small amount onto your stomach to keep the skin soft and pliable. You can also use it when dieting and losing weight. Stretch marks cannot be removed, but some will fade over time. I would suggest using this rich cream daily; it may seem a bit oily at first, but it is easily absorbed into your skin.

Mix together all ingredients except the vanilla extract. Heat the mixture gently until the cocoa butter and beeswax have melted; stir well.

Remove from the heat and stir in the vanilla extract, if desired. Allow to cool completely.

Store in a clean jar with a tight-fitting lid. Massage into your skin.

Yield: 3 ounces

The rose has become a symbol of beauty; its scent is unique and well known. No other flower is as regarded or used for as many cosmetic purposes as the rose. Shakespeare's Juliet proclaimed from her balcony in Verona, Italy, "A rose by any other name would smell as sweet." This lotion uses rose water, a wonderful skin softener with the lovely scent of roses.

Mix together the almond oil and beeswax and heat gently until the beeswax is melted. This can be done in a water bath, a double boiler, and even in the microwave if watched closely.

Slowly pour the rose water into the oil mixture. Stir well, and continue stirring off and on as it cools; it may seem thin at first, but it will turn into a lovely thick, white lotion. You may also pour the mixture into a blender or use a hand mixer.

Allow to cool completely, then store in a clean jar with a tight-fitting lid. Massage into your skin.

Yield: 4 ounces

Rose Lotion

¼ cup almond oil
1 tablespoon grated beeswax
¼ cup rose water

Facial Treatments

*I*n our world, the face is a critical part of communication — when we are happy, sad, surprised, or upset, it can be seen on our faces. Since it is the first thing many people notice about us, keeping the face looking its best is the smartest thing you can do for yourself. Clean, healthy skin will boost your confidence and raise your self-esteem. Because it is constantly exposed to the environment, the face also shows signs of aging before many other body parts. Proper care has been proven to aid in keeping skin looking and feeling younger.

A facial softens the skin, unclogs pores, and removes impurities. It also helps to replace lost moisture and soothe the skin. Masks are an important element in this process. Facial masks are some of the oldest known beauty treatments. The ancient Egyptians used mud and clay to remove dead skin cells and heal blemishes. During the early 1600s many European women experimented with milk and egg masks. Many other ingredients have been used since, such as fresh foods, flowers, and herbs, to cleanse and nourish the skin. I like the treatments because they are fun and easy, and they give me a boost when I am feeling tired. You can use facial masks every day, once a week, or whenever you feel your skin can use a special treat. (I have a girlfriend, Melinda, who lives in facial masks. I cannot remember a time in college when she opened the door to her room without having a mask on.)

Having a facial is also very relaxing because it requires that you remain quiet and calm for ten to twenty minutes — it's amazing how seldom we allow ourselves to do that! The psychological benefits of facial treatments definitely equal—if not exceed—their physical benefits. Another benefit is the almost limitless number of facial products you can create at home using fresh ingredients. Why go out and buy one commercial product when you already have the ingredients for a dozen in your kitchen?

The following recipes usually make enough for a single application. Unless you are sharing the products with a friend, I would suggest making only single applications. This way you will not have to worry about their spoiling and you will always have a fresh batch. Many of the recipes contain fresh foods such as eggs, so any leftover products should be kept in the refrigerator in a clean jar with a tight-fitting lid or in a container covered with plastic wrap. The average mask lasts about one to two weeks in the refrigerator, but always check your product before using it. Clay products tend to last longer than most and if they dry out, they can be revived by adding more pure water.

GIVE YOURSELF A GREAT FACIAL

1. *Wash* your face thoroughly, using a mild soap or cleansing cream.

2. *Clean* your face, using an astringent to remove any dead skin, soap, or cleansing cream residue.

3. *Nourish* your face using a facial mask. Cover the skin with a light, even coat, avoiding the area around your eyes; now *Relax*. Choose a mask with ingredients that are best for your skin type, i.e., dry or oily. Leave the mask on for 15 to 20 minutes. Try not to talk or move your face too much.

4. *Rinse* your face thoroughly, using tepid water, and pat dry.

5. *Steam* your face to clean out your pores, using a large bowl or sink full of hot water. If you want to add herbs to your water, you can. I would suggest chamomile for normal skin, peppermint for oily, and rosemary for dry skin types. Make a tent, using a large bath towel, and lean over the water for 10 to 15 minutes to open your pores.

6. *Rinse* thoroughly, starting with warm water then slowly changing to cold water to slowly clean and close the pores. (This is very important, especially if you are going outside.)

7. *Moisturize* your face with a light moisturizer. Massage the cream or lotion onto your face and allow it to soak in.

8. *Smile!* Your skin is really clean and you look great!

If you're in a hurry and feel you don't have time for a complete facial, give yourself a minifacial: Clean your face. Put on a simple, 1-ingredient mask (plain yogurt or avocado always works) for 5 to 10 minutes. Jump in the shower and rinse off the mask while opening your pores. Rinse your face with cool, clear water and moisturize.

Beauty Mayo

1¼ cups vegetable oil
1 teaspoon salt
1 egg
½ cup apple cider vinegar

*M*ayonnaise is an important ingredient in many natural beauty treatments. Regular commercial mayonnaise works well, but if you want to master the art of making mayonnaise and create your own, here is the perfect recipe. I call it "beauty mayo" because it contains everything you need for beautiful skin and hair: eggs, oil, and vinegar. You can use it alone as a face mask or as a recipe ingredient whenever mayonnaise is called for. It also makes a decent sandwich spread!

A blender or food processor really helps in this recipe. In a blender, mix ¼ cup oil, salt, and egg. With the blender on, slowly pour another ¼ cup oil, in a very thin stream, into the whirling mixture. Keep the blender mixing. Slowly pour into the whirling mixture half of the vinegar in a slow, steady stream. Keep the blender mixing. Slowly pour into the mixture another ¼ cup of oil followed by the rest of the vinegar. Continue blending.

Slowly add the rest of the oil. You should now have a thick, white, creamy mayonnaise. Remember, making mayonnaise is an art so you may need to practice, but once you master it you will never forget it.

Pour your mayonnaise into a clean container and store in the refrigerator. You can use this mixture in any recipe that calls for mayonnaise.

Yield: 16 ounces

Marie Antoinette Mask

Marie Antoinette, wife of King Louis XVI, may have been out of touch with reality and her subjects when she was quoted as saying, "If they don't have bread, let them eat cake!" There is no doubt, however, that she was a great beauty. Many believe that Marie Antoinette herself used this mixture to keep her skin clear and glowing. Today it is a popular facial treatment throughout France. It is suitable for all skin types, but because it does contain alcohol it can be drying. Be sure to moisturize your skin thoroughly afterward.

1 tablespoon cognac (or any alcohol will do)
1 egg
¼ cup nonfat dry milk powder
Juice of 1 lemon

Place all of the ingredients in a blender and mix well. If you do not want to use a blender, you can mix well by stirring with a fork or wire whisk.

Apply to your face and allow to dry, approximately 15 minutes.

Use remaining cream as a cleanser to remove the mask. Rinse your face thoroughly with warm water and pat dry.

Note: Any remaining mixture should be kept in the refrigerator.

Yield: approximately 2 ounces

Apricot Facial Mask

½ cup dried apricots
½ cup warm water
1 tablespoon nonfat dry milk powder
1 tablespoon honey

If your complexion has become colorless and dull, this mask can be used to revitalize it. Apricots are rich in vitamin A, which is important for healthy skin. Combined with milk and honey, they return moisture to the skin, helping it to look and feel smoother and softer. My daughter loves to eat any leftovers from this mask — it tastes great on toast!

Place all of the ingredients in the blender and blend until smooth.

Spread on your face and leave on for 15 minutes. Rinse off with tepid water and pat dry.

Yield: approximately 4 ounces

Country Garden Facial Mask

¼ cup grated carrot
1½ teaspoons mayonnaise (Use a commercial brand or the recipe for Beauty Mayo on page 94.)

The carrot is a featured vegetable in many country gardens. Carrots are an excellent source of beta-carotene, or provitamin A, which is important for healthy skin. Grated carrots hydrate the skin and help clear away dead cells. This is a rich mask that remains moist on the face.

Mix the carrot and mayonnaise together.

Spread on your face and leave on for 15 minutes. Rinse clean with tepid water and pat dry.

Yield: 2 ounces

Surprise-Party Facial Mask

*M*y girlfriend Nancy developed this mask when we were in high school. I will never forget the night I first used it. She talked me into covering my face with this pale green mask—then secretly invited over a group of our friends. I was so embarrassed I ran to her parents' bathroom and rinsed everything off. Today, I'm much less sensitive about people witnessing my beauty treatments, though this mask still gives my daughter a scare. This recipe is perfect for very dry skin because both the avocado and banana are rich in natural oils.

½ average-size avocado, mashed
½ ripe banana, mashed

Mix the avocado and banana together until smooth and creamy.

Spread on your face and leave on for 15 minutes. Rinse your face clean with tepid water and pat dry.

Yield: approximately 4 ounces

Old-Fashioned Oatmeal Masks

*O*atmeal comforts and nourishes the skin—it's rich in protein, potassium, iron, phosphates, magnesium, and silicon. It is perfect for individuals with sensitive skin because it is naturally gentle and mild. The three masks that follow offer an oatmeal mask for all skin types.

Mix all the ingredients together into a smooth paste.

Spread on your face and leave on for 15 minutes. Rinse your face clean with tepid water and pat dry.

Yield each mask: approximately 6 to 8 ounces

FOR OILY SKIN

½ cup cooked oatmeal
1 egg white
1 tablespoon fresh lemon juice
½ cup mashed apple

FOR DRY SKIN

½ cup cooked oatmeal
1 egg yolk
½ banana, mashed
1 tablespoon honey

FOR NORMAL SKIN

½ cup cooked oatmeal
1 whole egg
1 tablespoon almond oil

Beauty Queen Mask

In 1922 my grandmother was a princess in the Tournament of Roses parade in Pasadena, California. She remembers using eggs, honey, and almond oil as a mask to make her face soft and smooth. Her skin must have glowed as she waved to the crowds from her flower-covered float! I created this recipe after she told me this story—it is a rich moisturizing mask designed to nourish dry, flaky skin. Honey has natural antiseptic properties known to help in regenerating damaged skin tissues. Egg yolk contains lecithin, an antioxidant, like vitamin E, that acts as a natural preservative. After using this mask, your face should feel smoother and softer.

1 egg yolk
1 teaspoon honey
1 teaspoon almond oil
1 teaspoon vitamin E oil

Place all the ingredients together in a bowl and stir until smooth.

Spread on your face and leave on for 15 minutes. Rinse off with warm water and pat dry.

Yield: approximately 2 ounces

Natural Clay Masks

Clay or mud masks are some of the oldest natural beauty treatments still employed today. People have used the earth for centuries to deep cleanse the skin. Usually a wet mud is made by mixing naturally occurring clay with water, which is then applied to the face or the entire body. As this mud dries, it draws out oils, surface impurities, and dead skin cells, leaving the skin soft and smooth. Clay masks can also be used on the hair to deep cleanse and condition it. Remember: You never want to use earth directly from your yard these days, because it can contain harmful bacteria. It is best to purchase sterilized clay from your natural food store or pharmacy. See page 100 for a sampling of some of the more common clays you will find.

2 tablespoons natural clay
1–2 tablespoons distilled water

Fuller's earth: A fine gray clay that comes from algae found in seabeds and river bottoms.

Kaolin clay: Sometimes called "China Clay," this is a fine white powder originally obtained from Kaolin Hill in China.

French green clay: A fine, pale green clay that comes from southern France.

Bentonite: A volcanic white clay found in the midwestern United States and Canada.

Rhassoul mud: A red clay from the Atlas Mountains in North Africa.

Mix your clay mask fresh each time using equal parts clay and water. Stir well until you have a smooth paste.

To use: Spread the mixture on clean skin and leave on for 15 to 20 minutes, until dry. Rinse well with warm water followed by cool water and pat your skin dry.

Yield: 1 ounce, enough for one facial mask

Salsa Facial

I love salsa, and I put it on everything, even my face! This recipe is perfect for stressed-out or oily skin. Tomato, parsley, and cucumber are combined here to make a mildly acidic and astringent mask. Be careful not to use commercial salsa that contains peppers or spices, as this could cause discomfort and even breakouts on your face.

½ small tomato
¼ cup chopped cucumber (with peel)
2 tablespoons fresh parsley, chopped
1 teaspoon fresh lemon juice
1 egg white (optional)

Combine all of the ingredients except the egg white in a blender or food processor and purée. Stir in the egg white, if desired.

Apply to your face and leave on for 10 minutes. Rinse off with tepid water and pat dry. Refrigerate any leftover mask.

Yield: 4 ounces

Summer Watermelon Mask

Fresh watermelon is one of the simple pleasures of summer. It also makes a great toning facial mask. It contains a high amount of vitamins A, B, and C, all of which keep skin healthy and glowing. The consistency of this mask is thinner than most, and you may want to use a damp piece of cheesecloth or gauze over the mask to keep it on your face.

¼ cup watermelon, removed from the rind

Mash the fruit in a ceramic bowl, using a spoon or fork, until smooth (it should have the consistency of thin applesauce).

Spread the mixture on your face (make sure your skin is clean). Lie down and leave the mixture on your face for 20 minutes. If it seems to want to slide off, place a wet piece of cheesecloth or gauze over the watermelon to keep it in place.

Rinse well with cool water and pat dry.

Yield: 2 ounces

Mediterranean Mask

¼ cup mashed cooked chickpeas
1 teaspoon olive oil
¼ teaspoon fresh lemon juice
1 egg yolk

*C*hickpeas (garbanzo beans) contain a great deal of protein and make an excellent, nourishing facial mask. This recipe is similar to a favorite Mediterranean one for hummus. I have omitted the garlic, as it can be absorbed through the skin — you don't want to smell like garlic after a facial!

Mix together all ingredients into a smooth paste.

Spread over your face. Let dry for 20 minutes.

Rinse off with warm water followed by cold water. Pat your skin dry.

Yield: 3 ounces

Swiss Milkmaid Mask

¼ cup buttermilk
¼ cup powdered milk or powdered buttermilk

*I*n Switzerland, dairy products are well known for creating healthy skin and hair because they are rich in protein and vitamins. This mask is simple to make and the results are noticeable — it leaves my skin smooth and glowing. You may also use this mask on your hands and body for allover conditioning.

Mix together the buttermilk and powdered milk to form a smooth paste.

Spread an even layer of this milk paste over your face and neck. (I find that a small pastry brush or paintbrush gives me an even layer and does not pull the skin.) Leave the mask on your face until dry, 15 to 20 minutes.

Rinse off with cool water and pat your face dry. Store any leftover mask in the refrigerator, or share it with a friend.

Yield: 3 ounces

Swedish Rose Hip Mask

I *recently purchased at a used-book store a pamphlet written in 1966 entitled "Swedish Beauty Secrets." The number-one beauty secret of Swedish women was said to be rose hips. Rose hips are rich in vitamin C (they contain 40 percent more vitamin C than oranges) and make a facial mask that is perfect for clearing the skin of blemishes. Dried rose hips are easy to find and are in most natural food stores. If you have a rosebush in your yard, harvest the rose hips in the fall. Be sure to check your variety of rosebush, as not all produce rose hips.*

8–10 fresh or dried rose hips
¼ cup distilled water

If using dried rose hips: Place the rose hips in a ceramic container and cover with the water. Let soak until soft, a few hours or overnight. If using fresh rose hips: Place rose hips in a ceramic container and cover with the water. You do not need to let them soak.

Pour the mixture into a blender and blend until smooth. If you do not have a blender, mash the rose hips by hand until you have a smooth paste.

Spread on your face and leave on for 10 minutes. Rinse off with cool water and splash your face with rose water. Pat your skin dry.

Yield: 2 ounces

Brewer's Yeast Mask

1 teaspoon powdered brewer's yeast or
   6 tablets, crushed
1 tablespoon buttermilk or plain
   yogurt

Brewer's yeast was used by the early Greeks and Romans for a wide variety of medicinal purposes because it is an excellent source of protein, all of the B vitamins, and several minerals (it even contains gold). It is a by-product of beer, and is edible. It comes in powdered, liquid, or tablet form; many people take brewer's yeast as a dietary supplement (it does wonders for your hair and nails). It can be found in natural food stores.

Mix together the brewer's yeast and buttermilk until smooth.

Spread an even layer of this mixture over your face and neck. (I like to use a small pastry brush or paintbrush as it gives me an even layer and does not pull the skin.) Leave the mask on your face until dry, 10 to 20 minutes.

Rinse off the mask with cool water and pat your face dry. Store any leftover mask in the refrigerator.

Yield: 1 ounce

Gelatin masks are smooth and cool. They can be peeled off the face or easily rinsed away, removing dead skin cells. Using your favorite fruit or vegetable juice, they are easy and fun to make. After using one of these masks your face feels refreshed and new.

Combine the gelatin and fruit juice in a clean, oven-proof glass container. Heat gently to dissolve the gelatin completely. (Use a microwave oven for 45 seconds to 1 minute on High, or place in a double boiler on the stove top.)

Place the gelatin in the refrigerator and cool until almost set (about 30 minutes).

Spread a thin layer of the gelatin over your face and allow to dry. Peel off and rinse your face thoroughly with cool, clear water.

Yield: 4 ounces

Fruit Gel Masks

1 packet unflavored gelatin (about 1 tablespoon)
½ cup fruit juice (see following list)

Juices to try:

FOR NORMAL TO DRY SKIN

Apple, pear, peach, raspberry

FOR OILY SKIN

Tomato, grapefruit, lemon, white grape

SINGLE-INGREDIENT MASKS FROM
NATURE'S SKIN SALON

Avocado: Soften rough, dry skin with a mashed avocado. The unsaturated fatty acids of the alligator pear stimulate your skin's own natural production of oil (this is not for oily skin).

Egg: Eggs are great for your skin. The whites are very astringent and drying, and the yolks are rich in natural moisturizers. Egg yolks are a major source of lecithin, a natural emollient and preservative.

Plain yogurt: Rich in protein, calcium, and vitamins, yogurt makes an excellent mask for all skin types. Yogurt is easily absorbed into the skin and has super softening qualities.

Strawberries: I have a cousin in Germany who grows strawberries and makes herself a weekly strawberry mask. Strawberries contain salicylic acid (found in aspirin), which rids the skin of dead cells, allowing it to absorb moisture more efficiently.

Banana: Do you have overripe bananas in your fruit bowl? Instead of making muffins or bread, give yourself a nourishing facial mask. Bananas are great for dry skin because they are rich in potassium and vitamin A. They also contain no substances known to aggravate the skin.

Cucumber: Grated cucumbers make a gentle and mild astringent mask. It is especially soothing for sunburned skin.

Mayonnaise: Mayonnaise has it all—oil, eggs, and vinegar. It is naturally soothing to the skin, and improves skin texture. Mayonnaise is hard to beat for the conditioning power it provides.

Pear: Pears are a good source of sorbitol; other fruits that contain a high amount are apples, cherries, plums, and berries. Sorbitol is a humectant that gives a smooth feeling to your skin. Pears are especially soothing for red, blotchy skin. Apply either the fresh juice or the mashed fruit on your face.

Tomato: Tomatoes are effective on blackheads and oily skin. The juice of the tomato has astringent properties that help remove dead skin cells and deep-clean the skin's surface.

Piña Colada Mask

This fresh tropical mask will boost your complexion and give it a healthy glow. The key ingredient is fresh pineapple, which is rich in the enzyme bromelain. This active ingredient cleanses and freshens the skin by removing dead skin cells and other surface impurities. Coconut milk is easy to make yourself or you can purchase it canned at the grocery store. The canned option usually has extra sugar added, but that will not affect the outcome of the recipe.

¼ cup fresh, chopped pineapple
1 tablespoon coconut milk
2 teaspoons macadamia nut oil
  (optional for oily skin types)

Place all ingredients in a blender or food processor and blend until smooth.

To use: Spread the mixture in a thin layer over clean skin. Leave on for 5 to 10 minutes and then rinse well with warm water and pat skin dry.

Note: To make your own coconut milk. Place 1 cup fresh, grated coconut in a bowl and cover with 1 cup boiling water. Let sit until cool and then strain. The liquid is your coconut milk.

Yield: 3 ounces

Strawberry Acne Mask

½ cup fresh strawberries
1 egg white
2 teaspoons honey

Strawberries are rich in salicylic acid, the same key ingredient in many commercial acne products; honey is also a known antibacterial ingredient. Together they make a powerful facial treatment for troubled skin.

Mix together all ingredients until smooth, using a blender or a fork.

To use: Spread over your face and neck and let sit for 20 minutes. Rinse with cool water and pat your skin dry. Refrigerate any leftover mask and discard after one week.

Yield: 4 ounces

Fresh Carrot Mask

¼ cup fresh carrot juice, made from approximately 2 large carrots
¼ cup white kaolin clay or any natural clay

The orange-colored roots of the carrot plant are rich in vitamin A, often referred to as the "beauty" vitamin because of its importance in maintaining healthy skin and hair. Fresh carrot juice has strong antiseptic qualities, making it an excellent ingredient for a facial treatment for blemished skin. You may purchase fresh carrot juice, or make your own using a high-speed blender, food processor, or juice machine. For extremely dry skin, add 1 teaspoon of light oil to this recipe.

Mix together the carrot juice and clay until smooth. For a thicker mask you may add more clay.

To use: Spread the mixture on clean skin using your fingertips or a small brush. Let sit for 20 minutes, rinse well with warm water followed by cool, and pat the skin dry. Store any remaining mask in the refrigerator for up to one week.

Yield: 2 ounces, enough for one to two masks

ACNE OR TROUBLED SKIN CARE

If your skin tends to break out or you develop an acne problem, here are a few simple guidelines to keep in mind for a healthy, glowing complexion:

- Fight acne from the inside out by eating a balanced diet full of fiber, fresh vegetables, and fruits.

- Drink plenty of liquids to flush any impurities from the system—at least 12 glasses of water or water-based beverages, such as herbal tea or diluted fruit juices, daily.

- Chocolate and cola are fine, but avoid seafood and salty snacks. They are both sources of iodine, which can aggravate acne in some people.

- Take a well-balanced vitamin and mineral supplement. Vitamins A and B_6, zinc, and chromium help to clear up acne.

- Keep your fingers out of cosmetic products. Pour creams, lotions, and makeup into clean hands or use a small spoon to scoop them out. This will prevent you from introducing germs and bacteria in the products.

- Keep your hand off your face. Touching the face during the day will only irritate blemishes; plus it exposes the skin to harmful bacteria.

- An ounce of prevention is worth a pound of cure. Keep skin clean. Wash your face before going to bed at night and use a weekly scrub such as ground sunflower seeds, oatmeal, or cornmeal to keep pores clear.

- If your skin is broken out, do not steam your face in an effort to open up the pores. This can aggravate the condition by stimulating blood vessels and activating oil glands. Instead, apply hot towels to your face for no more than 1 minute.

- Get plenty of rest. Lack of sleep can cause stress and lead to unexpected breakouts. Remember a clear head equates to clear skin.

NATURAL EYE CARE

I get more questions from readers on eye care than any other subject. Puffiness, dark circles, wrinkles, and lash disasters all seem to top the list. Here are some natural cures and treatments to give you prettier eyes:

Puffiness: Under-eye puffiness can be caused by a variety of reasons: diet, allergies, or extra fluid in your system. To treat morning puffiness, follow these simple steps: Splash your face with very cold water. With a very light touch tap gently around your eyes to encourage fluids to move away from the eye area. Place a cold compress such as cucumber slices, tea bags, witch hazel pads, or potato slices over your eyes and relax for 15 to 20 minutes.

Crow's feet and wrinkles: Prevention is the name of the game in avoiding premature wrinkling around the eye area. Buy a good pair of sunglasses and wear them; they are your best beauty tools. Don't smoke; there are dozens of reasons not to, so add wrinkle prevention to the list. Also, avoid unnecessary stretching of the skin. Do not rub your eyes, and use a gentle eye makeup remover each evening.

Dark circles: The skin under the eyes is so thin that in some people the blood passing through the tiny veins near the surface shows through, giving the area a bluish or grayish cast or dark circles. Heredity, fatigue, and illness can all make under-eye circles more pronounced. Sleep and cosmetic camouflage are your two best treatments for dark circles. Make sure you get at least 8 hours of sleep each night.

Lush lashes: Hair, including your eyelashes, grows in cycles. An eyelash grows for about six months, then falls out or is pushed out by a new lash. Never rub your eyes, which could cause eyelash breakage. Instead, treat your lashes with castor oil or other light oils to keep them clean and conditioned.

Cooling Eye Gel

This cool, light gel is perfect for soothing and moisturizing tired eyes. Use it in the morning under makeup or at the end of the day for a quick pick-me-up. It contains fresh cucumber juice, aloe vera gel, and witch hazel, which are all naturally astringent and soothing.

Mix together the aloe vera, cucumber juice, and cornstarch. Heat until just boiling, but do not boil. This usually takes 1 minute on High in the microwave. Remove from your heat source and mix in the witch hazel. Stir well and allow the mixture to cool completely. You should have a clear, jellylike cream. Spoon into a small clean jar.

To use: Dab a small amount into the skin under your eyes, being careful not to rub or pull this delicate skin.

Yield: 1 ounce

1 tablespoon aloe vera gel
1 teaspoon fresh cucumber juice, strained
¼ teaspoon cornstarch
1 tablespoon witch hazel

Lip Treatments

*L*ip care products were some of the first cosmetic products used. Lip paints made by the Mesopotamians date back to 3500 B.C. In New England, Puritan women frowned on the use of cosmetics in general. However, they made lip balm recipes out of crushed rose petals to soothe and color their lips. In Paris in 1910 lipstick as we know it today was first introduced. It is now the most commonly used and purchased cosmetic product in the world.

Lip gloss and lip balms are a vital part of your beauty collection. They are also a cinch to create. The majority are made by simply melting together two or three ingredients. I like to use lip glosses under and over lipstick, as many lipsticks can be slightly drying. If you spend a lot of time outdoors or in the sun, you should always put sun protection on your lips.

Some of my friends brush their lips with a soft toothbrush to remove dead skin and keep them soft and smooth. I have found that a coating of natural oil such as coconut or almond and rubbing your lips gently with a warm washcloth also works well and is easier on the lips. Follow up with a fresh coat of lip gloss and your lips should glow with natural color!

Lip glosses and balms have a long shelf life and will last for at least a year. The products contained in this chapter require the general care and storage guidelines found on page 8.

Aloe Vera Lip Gloss

Aloe vera makes a soothing lip gloss with a very high moisture content. I like to use this gloss in the summer after my lips have spent time in the sun.

1 teaspoon aloe vera gel
½ teaspoon coconut oil
1 teaspoon petroleum jelly (optional)

Mix together all three ingredients in a shallow dish or cup using the back of a teaspoon. Gently heat the mixture until the coconut oil has melted. (I do this in the microwave on High for 30 seconds to 1 minute.) Pour the melted mixture into a lip gloss container or clean pillbox (both available at drugstores).

Cool completely, until the mixture is cool to the touch and solid. This takes about 10 to 20 minutes. You can speed up the cooling time by using the refrigerator.

Rub into your lips and enjoy.

Yield: ½ ounce

Almond and Cocoa Butter Lip Gloss

This lip gloss is good by itself or under lipstick. Cocoa butter conditions and protects the lips and has a mild chocolate scent. I like to use this gloss over lipstick for extra shine.

½ teaspoon grated beeswax
1 teaspoon cocoa butter (You may want to grate if using solid cocoa butter.)
1 teaspoon almond oil

Melt the wax, cocoa butter, and oil together over medium heat in a glass measuring cup in a pan of boiling water (water-bath technique). Pour the melted mixture into a lip gloss container or clean pillbox (both available at drugstores).

Cool completely, until cool to the touch and solid in form. You can refrigerate the mixture to speed up cooling time.

Rub into your lips and enjoy.

Yield: ½ ounce

Flavored Coconut Lip Gloss

This is a supersimple and effective lip gloss that combines coconut oil with your favorite flavoring. Coconut oil is especially good for dry, cracked lips, as it helps lock in moisture. Flavored oils are easily found at the grocery store or gourmet cooking shops because they are used in candy making.

1 tablespoon coconut oil
Few drops flavored oil such as strawberry, orange, or coconut
Or
⅛ teaspoon flavored extract such as vanilla, peppermint, or almond

Mix ingredients well in a small dish with the back of a teaspoon. Spoon the mixture into a lip gloss container.

To use: Rub into your lips and enjoy.

Yield: approximately ½ ounce

Coconut-Almond Lip Gloss

This is a solid, waxy gloss that can even be formed into a lipstick. You can purchase empty lipstick containers or use old ones that have been cleaned out. Pour the melted gloss into these containers and allow to cool completely.

1 teaspoon coconut oil
1 teaspoon almond oil
½ teaspoon grated beeswax

Mix together the coconut oil, almond oil, and beeswax. Melt the ingredients in either the microwave for 1 to 2 minutes on High (watch closely) or place the mixture in a double boiler or water bath on the stove top.

Pour into a clean lip gloss container and cool completely, approximately 20 minutes.

Rub into your lips and enjoy.

Yield: approximately ½ ounce

Vanilla Lip Gloss

1 tablespoon grated beeswax
½ tablespoon coconut oil
⅛ teaspoon vitamin E oil
⅛ teaspoon pure vanilla extract

Pure vanilla extract gives this lip gloss a lovely scent and caramel color, not to mention a delicious flavor. Coconut oil, beeswax, and vitamin E oil preserve your lips by providing a protective layer that conditions and locks in moisture.

Place the beeswax, coconut oil, and vitamin E oil in an ovenproof container. Heat gently until the wax and oils are melted. Stir in vanilla extract and mix well. Pour the mixture into a clean container and allow it to cool completely. Rub onto lips with a clean finger or lip brush.

Yield: 1½ ounces

Chocolate Lip Gloss

1½ teaspoons grated cocoa butter
½ teaspoon coconut oil
⅛ teaspoon vitamin E oil
¼ teaspoon grated chocolate or 3 small
   chocolate chips (I like to use milk
   chocolate ones.)

From the colorful fruits of the cacao tree come the raw ingredients for chocolate. The two main substances obtained from the wrinkly pods are cocoa butter and unsweetened chocolate (sold as bitter chocolate or baking chocolate). This lip gloss, made from blending together cocoa butter and chocolate, is an excellent lip conditioner with a mildly sweet taste.

In a double boiler or the microwave oven, heat the cocoa butter, coconut oil, and vitamin E oil gently until melted. Stir in the chocolate and keep stirring until melted and well blended. Pour into a small lip gloss container and allow to cool completely.

To use: Spread on lips with a clean fingertip or lip brush.

Yield: ½ ounce

Castor Oil Lip Balm

Castor oil mixed with lanolin is soothing to dry, cracked lips and gives your lips a natural shine. I also use this recipe on my eyebrows to condition them and keep them in place.

Melt the castor oil, lanolin, and beeswax together over medium heat in a glass measuring cup in a pan of boiling water (water-bath technique).

Pour the melted mixture into a lip gloss container or clean pillbox (both available at drugstores). Cool completely, until cool to the touch, approximately 20 minutes.

Rub into your lips and enjoy.

Yield: ½ ounce

1 teaspoon castor oil
1 teaspoon lanolin or coconut oil
1 teaspoon grated beeswax

Beeswax Lipsticks

These are super little sticks to keep with you and use throughout the day, either alone or under your favorite lipstick. I also rub a bit on my heels at night to keep them soft (of course, not the same stick I use on my lips). Use them anywhere you can use a little extra conditioning.

Mix together all the ingredients in an ovenproof container. Heat the mixture gently in the microwave for 1 to 2 minutes on High or in a double boiler or water bath on the stove top, until everything is melted and you have a pale golden liquid.

Pour the melted mixture into a shallow greased pan or cardboard box lined with foil. (I use empty tea boxes.) Allow the mixture to cool, then cut into lipsticks.

¼ cup grated beeswax
3 tablespoons vegetable shortening
2 tablespoons cocoa butter
1 tablespoon light oil (I use almond oil.)

Store in a closed container or wrap each stick individually. These make nice gifts, especially in the winter months when your friends' lips may need some T.L.C. (tender loving care).

Rub the sticks over your lips.

Yield: 4 ounces, 10 to 12 sticks

Lip Stains

2 tablespoons almond oil
1 tablespoon grated beeswax
⅛ to 1 teaspoon beet juice or beetroot
 powder

Lip stains are perfect for giving your lips sheer, natural color. Carmine and alkanet root are popular natural pigments. Carmine is a red pigment derived from dried female cochineal insects. Alkanet root is also red and comes from a tree that grows in the Mediterranean region. I prefer using beets and beetroot powder because they're easier to find than carmine and alkanet root—and they're a better buy. Beetroot powder is a lovely purple-red color that is perfect for lip glosses. It has a sweet taste and is often used in place of sugar when cooking. All of the recipes in this chapter may be colored with beet juice or beetroot powder; you can experiment with the amounts to achieve different shades. If you are lucky enough to have fresh beets, you can easily make your own juice by blending or mashing the root and stem and straining out any solids.

Mix together the oil and wax and heat gently to melt the wax. The mixture may be heated in the microwave on High for 1 to 2 minutes or on the stove top using a double boiler or water bath.

Add the beet juice or powder and stir the mixture well. Do not worry if the mixture seems to separate; it will stay together when cool. As the mixture cools, you may add more juice or powder until you have the shade of color you desire, from pink to red.

Place in a clean container and apply to your lips with a clean finger or lip brush.

Note: You may also add the beet juice to the oil before melting the wax and then heat the mixture together—it won't separate as much. The results are the same when cool.

Yield: 1 ounce

Chapped Lip Cure

This is a treatment that has been passed down in my family for generations. My grandmother grew up in Ohio, where the winter weather is extremely cold and harsh. She remembers using this old-fashioned overnight cure for chapped lips. I use it year round because it works!

½ teaspoon glycerine or honey
½ teaspoon fresh lemon juice
½ teaspoon castor oil

Mix together all ingredients. Spread the mixture on your lips and leave on overnight. In the morning awake to smooth, soothed lips.

Any extra should be stored in the refrigerator because it contains fresh lemon juice, which can spoil.

Yield: ½ ounce

LUSCIOUS LIPS

Keep your lips looking and feeling their best with these simple tips. Lips are a unique part of our body in both appearance and construction. They have no sweat glands, few sebaceous oil glands, and their only protection from the outside world is saliva—which isn't really all that helpful.

- To gently exfoliate dry lips, cover them with a layer of light oil and, using a warm, wet washcloth, gently brush your lips, removing the dry skin. Some people use a soft toothbrush in place of the washcloth.

- Try to avoid licking your lips; this actually dries them out more, causing them to chap and crack.

- Condition your lips at night while you sleep by coating them with a layer of lip gloss or natural oil such as coconut oil before going to bed. Awake to soft, kissable lips.

- If you are susceptible to cold sores, look for products and recipes that contain peppermint or eucalyptus oil, which contain natural antimicrobials that are effective in fighting cold sores. You can also add a few drops of these oils to your favorite lip product recipe.

- If you spend a great deal of time outdoors, you should also use a commercial sunscreen on your lips, which are vulnerable to developing skin cancer if not protected from the sun's harmful UV rays.

Hydrotherapy: Shower and Bath Treatments

*H*ydrotherapy—using water to heal and relax the body—is a very ancient practice. Hippocrates, the father of medicine, praised the use of water and its benefits for the human body. Today many health spas are adding hydrotherapy treatments to their regimens. You can very easily create these treatments at home. The hot/cold shower is very popular today: take a hot shower for three minutes and then turn the water to cold for twenty seconds, then back to hot. This is believed to energize the body and improve circulation.

Whether you prefer a shower or a bath, you can treat yourself to skin-softening routines at home. Throughout history many great beauties have used bathing as a major part of their beauty routines. Helen of Troy took vinegar baths; Mary, Queen of Scots, bathed in wine; and we all know that Cleopatra was famous for her milk baths. Bathwater should be warm—90 to 100 degrees Fahrenheit is ideal (use a thermometer if necessary). A bath taken with water temperatures over 100 degrees can be more harmful than helpful to your body. Water that is too hot dilates tiny blood capillaries that can burst, making red marks on the skin. It also dries out the skin and makes you feel very tired.

This chapter contains natural beauty treatments for both the bath and shower. I tend to take showers; however, some of my favorite treatments are baths. I like the change in routine that a bath provides, and it allows me to really relax and unwind.

Many of the recipes in this chapter are for a single treatment. For these bath products, follow the general care and storage guidelines found on page 8.

Morning Wake-up!

I have found this treatment to be better than a cup of coffee in the morning. It is also a great cure for jet lag. I never travel without a small vial of peppermint oil.

2 cups sparkling mineral water or seltzer water
Juice of one lemon
2–3 drops peppermint oil (You could also use eucalyptus or camphor oil.)

Mix all of the ingredients together in a bowl.

While in the shower or bath after you have washed yourself, but before the final rinse, sponge this mixture all over your body, from head to toe (including your hair). Rinse off with tepid water (not too hot) and pat your skin dry.

Note: I love to use a big fluffy natural sea sponge, but you can also use a washcloth if a sponge is not available.

Yield: 16 ounces, 1 treatment

Pineapple Body Seltzer

The inspiration for this treatment came during my honeymoon in Hawaii, where fresh pineapple is abundant. Pineapple cleanses and freshens the skin. It contains bromelain, a protein-digesting enzyme that removes any dead skin cells, surface dirt, and oils, a process so necessary for healthy skin. This is a rejuvenating shower treatment and a great way to start the day. Be sure to moisturize well afterward, especially if you have dry or sensitive skin.

¼ fresh pineapple, puréed in a food processor or blender until smooth and creamy—about 1 cup (You can also substitute fresh pineapple juice if you wish.)
2 cups seltzer water or sparkling mineral water

Mix together the pineapple and seltzer water.

Use as a final rinse in the shower after you have finished washing. Use a clean natural sea sponge (or washcloth), and squeeze the pineapple water all over your skin and hair.

Rinse well with warm water, making sure you remove all the pineapple water. Pat yourself dry with a clean, fluffy towel and moisturize your skin all over.

Note: This is an excellent treatment for oily skin or acne. You may want to keep a small amount for a skin freshener—it's just as effective after the seltzer water goes flat!

Yield: 24 ounces, 1 treatment

Vinegar-Herb Bath

This slightly acidic bath helps to rinse away soap residues on your skin and reinstates your own natural acid balance. It is also a good way to counteract vaginal yeast infections because the acidic environment will kill many harmful organisms. This particular combination of herbs is guaranteed to alleviate stress. A vinegar bath is also an excellent way to use all of those gourmet herb vinegars you have been given as gifts. I once received a gorgeous bottle of raspberry vinegar that was excellent on salads, but was even more delightful in the bath!

1 cup apple cider vinegar
1 cup water
1 tablespoon fresh (or 1 teaspoon dried) rosemary
1 tablespoon fresh (or 1 teaspoon dried) tarragon
1 tablespoon fresh (or 1 teaspoon dried) mint leaves
1½ teaspoons fennel seeds

Combine all the ingredients and heat just until boiling. This can be done on the stove top or in the microwave for 1 to 2 minutes. Allow the mixture to steep for several hours or even overnight.

Strain off all solids by pouring the mixture through a fine strainer or through a coffee filter into a jar.

Pour the entire mixture into a warm bath and enjoy.

Note: This recipe can be doubled or tripled if you would like to have extra on hand. It also makes a great gift in a pretty colored bottle with a fresh sprig of rosemary or mint.

Yield: 18 ounces, enough for 1 bath

Cleopatra Milk Bath

1 tablespoon dried rosemary
1 tablespoon dried thyme
1 tablespoon dried mint
Peel of 1 orange
Peel of 1 lemon
2 cups boiling water
1 small (9.6 ounces) box dried milk, enough to make 3 quarts; if you have oily skin use nonfat milk powder

Even though no one knows exactly what Cleopatra looked like, there is no doubt that her beauty was very influential and captivating—especially for Julius Caesar and Marc Antony. One of her greatest beauty secrets was her milk bath. With this recipe you can enjoy a milk bath like Cleopatra in your own home and feel like the queen of the Nile.

Combine the herbs and citrus peels in a large ceramic bowl. Pour the boiling water over the herbs and peels and allow to steep for several hours (even overnight).

Strain off the liquid, removing all solids. Add the milk powder to this solution.

Draw a warm (not hot) bath and pour the entire mixture into the bath water. Soak in the tub for at least 20 minutes, or as long as you like.

Rinse the milk off your skin with warm water. You don't want it to sour on your skin, creating an unpleasant smell. Pat dry and moisturize your body.

Yield: approximately 16 ounces, enough for 1 bath

ural Beauty at Home

Super Muscle-Soothing Bath

This is the perfect bath after a day of strenuous physical activity. You can feel your muscles relaxing while you bathe. I keep a jar of this mixture in my bathroom and add a scoop or two to the bath after an especially grueling day. This treatment can be drying to your skin, so remember to moisturize thoroughly afterward.

1 cup salt
1 cup baking soda
1 cup epsom salts

Mix all ingredients together.

Start filling your bathtub with warm water. Pour the mixture into the bath slowly, allowing the minerals to dissolve completely. Step into the bath and *relax*.

Yield: 24 ounces, enough for 1 bath

HERB BATHS

Herb baths are easy to prepare and are also an excellent way to practice aromatherapy, using the scents to transform your mental state. The following is a list of popular herbs and their effects—experiment with different ones in combination. They can be added directly to the bathwater; however, if you're like me and hate to clean the tub, I suggest putting your herbs in a mesh bag (I like to use old nylon stockings). Simply place 1 cup of dried herbs or 2 cups of fresh into the stocking and knot the end, then tie this bag under the water faucet while you draw your bath. I have a girlfriend who uses a tea ball to hold her herbs, and is equally pleased with the results.

(continued)

Basil: Stimulates the memory, relieves stress, and cures depression

Bergamot: Cures depression

Chamomile: Relaxes and calms the nerves

Lavender: Relaxes and calms the nerves; good for babies

Marjoram: Relieves stress and relaxes

Mint: Uplifts the spirit and energizes

Rosemary: Stimulates the memory

Sage: Invigorates the body

Northwest Pine Bath

1 cup pine needles
2 cups water

The smell of pine produces a feeling of serenity and peacefulness. This is a very gentle and relaxing bath. If you do not live in the northwest, where pine trees are abundant, you can produce a year's supply of baths by boiling the needles (it's all right if they are a little dry) from your Christmas tree.

Place the pine needles in a large pot on the stove and cover with the water. Bring the water to a boil and remove the pan from the heat.

Allow the pine water to cool completely, about 30 minutes.

Strain off the pine needles and discard. Pour the clear, pine-scented water into a clean bottle. Add 2 cups of this pine water to your bathwater.

Yield: 16 ounces, enough for 1 bath

Rose Floral Bath

The rose is one of the oldest flowers. It has been grown for more than five thousand years in the ancient gardens of west Asia and northeast Africa. The rose signifies love, and the rosebud represents beauty and youth. Many aromatherapists value the scent of the rose for its calming effects—it is especially effective for relieving tension in women. If you have received a special bouquet of roses and cannot bear to throw them out, use the petals to prepare this simple but special bath.

2 cups rose water
2 cups rose petals, or as many as you
    want to use
2–3 drops rose oil (optional)

Draw yourself a nice warm bath. Pour in the rose water, and rose oil, if desired, and scatter the rose petals on top of the water.

Climb in and enjoy the scent and feel of the rose petals as you relax.

Yield: 16 ounces, enough for 1 bath

Oatmeal Cookie Bath

1 cup oatmeal
1 cup warm water
1 tablespoon vanilla extract
½ cup baking soda

Baking cookies is one of my daughter's favorite activities. If you've eaten a fresh oatmeal cookie, you know how good they can taste. Like warm cookies, this bath is comforting and relaxing, and smells delicious. I like to fix myself a cup of warm milk to enjoy in the tub while bathing. Oatmeal is soothing to dry, itchy skin because it is rich in protein and B vitamins.

Combine all the ingredients together in a blender or food processor. Blend on high speed until you have a smooth paste.

Pour this paste under the running water while drawing the bath. Step into the tub and enjoy.

Yield: 8 ounces, enough for 1 bath

Colored Bath Salts

1 cup epsom salts
¼ cup kosher salt or sea salt, coarsely ground (available in many grocery stores)
Food coloring
Essential oils, such as peppermint, coconut, or bitter orange (optional)

Bath salts are a lot of fun to make and use because you can choose the colors and scents to add to the salts. I like to fill a pretty glass jar with alternating colors of bath salts to keep in my bathroom or give as gifts. Adding your favorite scent also adds to the bath experience. Last Christmas, I gave many of my friends red and white "peppermint" bath salts that smelled just like candy canes. Another of my favorites is a coconut-scented blue bath salt I have named Blue Hawaii, after my favorite Elvis Presley movie.

Mix together the epsom salts and kosher salt. Add a few drops of your favorite color and stir well to blend. (Blue and green are pretty shades to use.) If you would like to scent your bath salts, add a few drops of the essential oils.

Pour the salts into a container with a lid or into a resealable plastic bag and close tightly. When you are drawing a bath, add about ¼ cup of these bath salts under the running water.

Note: You may substitute cornstarch or baking soda for the kosher salt in this recipe.

Yield: 10 ounces

Old-Fashioned Bubble Bath

For a totally indulgent treat, it's hard to beat a good old-fashioned bubble bath. An instant mood enhancer, nothing can make you feel as good as being surrounded by millions of rich, creamy white bubbles. This is a recipe my grandmother used to make for me, and I never wanted to get out of the tub.

½ cup mild liquid soap
1 tablespoon sugar or honey
1 egg white

Mix together all of the ingredients and pour the entire mixture under the running water as you draw your bath.

Note: You may want to add a little of your favorite oil to the bath for extra skin conditioning.

Yield: 6 ounces, enough for one bubble bath

Scrubbing Sacks

These are fun little bundles to have around the bathroom. Using them keeps your skin soft and clean. Make up extras to tuck into gift baskets for friends. The basic directions for making the sacks are the same—vary the ingredients for different effects and individuals. I use gauze squares found in the first-aid section of the grocery store, but any fine-meshed material will work. I like to tie up the sacks with pretty ribbon or string (make sure it is waterproof).

1 large gauze square (4 × 4 inches)
   or cheesecloth
1 tablespoon dried herbs or 3
   tablespoons fresh (see list below)
½ cup grated soap flakes
½ cup oatmeal
3–4 drops essential oil
1 6-inch piece cotton string

WAKE-UP SACK

Peppermint, oatmeal, soap, and
   peppermint oil

RELAXING SACK

Chamomile, oatmeal, soap, and
   lavender oil

FOR WOMEN ONLY

Rose hips, oatmeal, soap, and rose oil

FOR MEN ONLY

Sage, oatmeal, soap, and rosemary oil

Unfold the gauze square and lay flat.

Mix together the herbs, soap, oatmeal, and essential oil. Place the soap mixture on the gauze square, and using the string, tie up the corners, creating a little pouch or sack. Use this sack in the bath or shower for scrubbing your skin clean. Hang it to dry between uses and it will last longer.

Note: Experiment with your own favorite mix of herbs and oils.

*W*alk into any natural beauty boutique and you will find a variety of effervescent bath bombs to purchase. They have become almost as popular as scented bath salts and bubble baths. What is a bath bomb? It is a combination of baking soda and citric acid that, when added to your bath, explodes into a fit of bubbles. They are fun to use and just as much fun to make. You can get creative with scents and colors for your bath creations as well as using candy molds for fun shapes. Citric acid powder can be found at many natural food stores, or you may use powdered vitamin C. I have also seen these powders which are used in canning fruits in the grocery store.

Place all of the dry ingredients into a bowl and mix well. Add the oil to the dry mixture and blend until you have a soft dough. Add fragrance and color if you desire. Shape the dough into small balls and place on a sheet of waxed paper. Let the bath bombs harden and dry; this usually takes 24 to 48 hours.

To use: Drop one to three bombs into a warm bath and enjoy!

Yield: 4 ounces, enough for 6 bath bombs, depending on size

Fizzing Bath Bombs

2 tablespoons citric acid powder

2 tablespoons cornstarch

¼ cup baking soda

3 tablespoons light oil such as canola, almond, or sunflower

3–6 drops essential oil or fragrance oil (optional)

2–3 drops food coloring (optional)

Mustard Bath

½ cup baking soda
2 tablespoons powdered mustard
2 drops essential oil of rosemary
2 drops essential oil of eucalyptus or
 tea tree oil

*I*n England, mustard baths are very popular. They're said to relieve stress, muscle soreness, and sleeplessness. The warmth of the mustard helps open the pores, allowing you to sweat out any impurities. This recipe can also be used as a footbath.

Mix together all ingredients and pour into a clean, dry container.

To use: Add ¼ cup to the bath under running water. After your bath, dress warmly until your pores are fully closed.

For a footbath: Add 1 tablespoon of the bath powder to a basin of hot water, then soak your feet for 15 minutes.

Yield: 5 ounces, enough for 2 baths

Foaming Bath Salts

½ cup liquid soap
1 tablespoon light oil
Food coloring (optional)
6 cups rock salt or kosher salt

*A*ny bath salt recipe can be made to "foam" by adding liquid soap to it. You get the benefits of bath salts with the pleasure of bubbles. What could be better? These bubbling bath salts are perfect for gift giving and can be scented to match individual tastes.

Mix together the soap, oil, and food coloring. Pour this mixture over the rock salt in a large bowl. Stir completely until the salt crystals are evenly coated.

Spread the salts out in a thin layer on a cookie sheet covered with wax paper and allow the mixture to air-dry. This can take up to 24 hours. Sometimes to speed up the process I put the salts in the oven on the lowest setting and check it every couple of hours. You want all of the moisture to evaporate, leaving you with dry salts.

To use: Pour ¼ cup of the salts into a warm bath under the running water and enjoy.

Yield: 48 ounces, enough for 24 baths

Relaxing Lavender Bath

This recipe contains lavender, as a relaxant, as well as oatmeal and baking soda, which are soothing to dry, sensitive skin. It also has healing properties, which makes it an ideal bath for calming a bad rash, sunburn, or insect bites.

1 cup dried lavender flowers
2 cups oatmeal
½ cup baking soda

Place all the ingredients inside a food processor or blender. Grind until you have a smooth, fine powder. The powder should have the consistency of whole-grain flour. Pour into a clean airtight container or a resealable plastic bag.

To use: Pour ½ cup into your bath as you fill the tub.

Yield: 28 ounces, enough for 7 baths

CREATING THE ULTIMATE BATH ENVIRONMENT

Add to your bathing experience by creating a wonderful bath environment that will please all of your senses.

Sound: Place a small stereo inside your bathroom (a safe distance from the tub) and play your favorite sing-along songs, nature sounds, or classical music. Hang a wind chime outside your window and let the gentle breeze entertain you.

Color: Color is visible light energy, and it can be used almost anywhere to create or enhance your mood. Tint your bathwater using a few drops of food coloring. Red for power, orange for independence, yellow for soothing your nerves, green for harmony, blue for serenity, and violet for creativity.

Lighting: Candlelight has become extremely popular in the bath. It is soothing and relaxing. Install a dimmer on your light switch so that you can control the light level of the room.

Poetry: Reading in the bath is as popular as ever. Choose a favorite poem, quotation, or book to focus on.

Temperature: The temperature of the bath is very important since it can affect your energy level and mood. A warm bath set at body temperature is an instant energizer, whereas a hot bath will help you sleep at night.

Flowers: Bring a bit of nature indoors. Place a bouquet of fresh flowers in your bath for beauty and fragrance.

Refreshments: In the morning, enjoy a cool drink of iced mineral water. In the evening, a cup of warm herbal tea is very soothing.

After bath: Continue the mood of your bath by using your fluffiest cotton towel, scented powder, and after-bath splash. Get dressed to music, or snuggle into a warm bed and finish that book.

Body Treatments

*O*ur skin has three important functions: to protect the body from the environment, to enhance our sense of feel, and to regulate the body's temperature. The skin is one of the largest organs of the body — the average person has more than three thousand square inches of surface area.

The body treatments in this chapter are wonderful for really caring for yourself and your skin, and they're also a great way to relax. Once a month I like to turn my home into a health spa, using one or two of these treatments to really pamper myself. You can also invite a special friend or loved one to share in your beauty "retreat."

Many of the treatments in this chapter exfoliate, or remove dead skin cells and impurities from the skin. This is very important for healthy and glowing skin all over the body because it allows the skin to retain more moisture. It also allows new skin to appear.

The majority of the recipes are for one application, but they can be doubled if you wish. The general care and storage guidelines found on page 8 should be followed. Any leftover products that contain fresh foods should always be refrigerated; they should be discarded after a week.

Salt Rub

2 cups kosher salt (or any coarse
   salt)
1 cup almond oil (or coconut,
   avocado, or olive oil)

This recipe is a favorite today at many exclusive health spas. Salt rubs are not a new treatment; they've been used for centuries by many civilizations. Coarse salt added to oil and massaged into your skin removes dead surface cells and dirt while simultaneously lubricating the skin. Never use this treatment on your face or on skin that has broken out, as it could be very irritating.

Mix the salt and oil together until it forms a thick paste.

While in the tub or shower, take a handful of the paste and massage it into your skin, starting with your feet (be careful, as the oil will make your feet very slippery). Massage the paste all over your body.

When you have finished and your body is covered, rinse off with warm water and pat dry. Do not use soap or you will remove the oil and spoil the moisturizing effect.

Save any extra paste in a clean container for your next treatment. It will keep for 1 to 2 months and does not need refrigeration.

Yield: 16 ounces

Raw Sugar Scrub

Raw sugar is perfect for freshening and moisturizing the skin. Sugar is quickly replacing salt as the scrub of choice in many top spas as it is not as dehydrating and can be used by all skin types. Body scrubs are helpful because they stimulate your circulation. A gentle rubdown can counteract stress, help rid the body of excess fluid, and really energize your whole system. I like to use raw sugar in this recipe for its coarse texture and subtle molasses scent. If you have oily skin, you should reduce the amount of walnut oil called for in this recipe — or leave it out completely.

1 cup raw sugar or granulated sugar
¼ cup walnut oil or light oil
½ teaspoon vitamin E oil

Mix together all the ingredients in a large glass or ceramic bowl. Spoon into a clean jar with a tight-fitting lid.

To use: Massage a tablespoon or two all over your body to gently exfoliate and moisturize your skin. Store any remaining scrub in a cool, dry location. You may need to stir the product between uses.

Yield: 10 ounces, enough for 4 to 5 full-body treatments

EXFOLIATION

The three most important things you can do for your skin are clean it, moisturize it, and protect it from the sun. Exfoliation helps to deep cleanse your skin, which will help it retain more moisture and look fresher, younger, and healthier.

Regular removal of dead skin cells and surface impurities or exfoliation helps prevent excessive thickening of your skin, which makes it appear sallow or pasty—not very attractive.

There are several methods of skin exfoliators you can use. For your facial skin you can use a cotton washcloth, complexion brush, or facial scrub such as sugar or ground oatmeal. Use gentle circular strokes and do not work on any one area for too long, which can be irritating. You can exfoliate as often as your skin can take it—for most people this is weekly. For your body you can use stronger scrubs and brushes such as loofah sponges, body brushes, and salt or sugar rubs. For classic rough skin areas such as feet, knees, and elbows you may use a natural pumice stone.

Use care when scrubbing your skin and a bit of common sense; never exfoliate if your skin is broken out or sore. If excessive redness or irritation develops, cut back or stop completely for a few days and switch to a gentler method.

Herbal Body Wrap

In European health spas, women pay dearly for these wraps. They are believed to produce miraculous results, such as weight loss and cellulite removal. Though this has yet to be proven, you will probably lose some water weight, and it is a great way to relax totally. You will need a partner's help for this treatment when wrapping yourself up.

Fill a large sink or bucket with very hot (but not boiling) water. Pour in your herbs and allow to steep for 5 minutes. Add the beach towel or sheets.

Lay the plastic drop cloth on your bed. Wring out the towel or sheets and wrap around your body. Lie down on the bed and have your partner help you wrap yourself in the plastic drop cloth. Cover yourself with blankets and lie quietly for 10 minutes—no more. Don't overdo it. Try not to talk or be distracted.

Slowly unwrap yourself and get up. Enjoy the wonderful sense of relaxation this treatment provides!

Yield: 1 wrap

1 cup of your favorite herb or combination of herbs (I like to use chamomile, rosemary, lavender, and sage.)
Large beach towel or cotton sheets
Plastic drop cloth or shower curtain (Drop cloths can be found at hardware stores.)

Sea Mud Body Mask

This is a rich clay body mask that removes toxins from the skin and renews it. Kelp, aloe vera gel, and pure clay combine to give your whole body a healthy, radiant glow. Powdered kelp can be found in most natural food stores.

Mix together all ingredients until a smooth paste or mud is formed.

Spread the mud all over your face and body. (A medium-sized paintbrush is helpful in evenly spreading the mud over your body.) Allow the mud to dry for 15 to 20 minutes.

½ cup powdered clay
¼ cup powdered kelp
½ cup aloe vera gel
¼ cup seawater (If not available, mix sea salt with distilled water.)

Shower off with tepid water and pat dry. Use a rich moisturizer such as cocoa butter or coconut oil, as this treatment can be drying for certain skin types.

Note: If you do not want to cover your whole body in sea mud, you can do just your upper torso. Kelp powder alone makes a mineral-rich body scrub for removing surface impurities.

Yield: 12 ounces, enough for 1 treatment

Tropical Body Polish

I am mad about mangoes and delighted to find that they are now available in many grocery stores year round. These funny-looking fruits with the huge pits are chock-full of vitamins, and make the perfect treat for tired skin. After polishing your body with this recipe, your skin glows and is extremely smooth and soft.

1 whole mango
1 tablespoon ground avocado pit
   (see page 40)
1 tablespoon dried orange zest (the
   colored part of the peel)

Remove the peel and seed from the mango and mash the fruit. Stir in the ground avocado pit and orange zest.

Use the mixture as an allover body treatment while showering, to exfoliate and moisturize your skin. Take a small amount of the scrub in your hand and rub well into your damp skin; repeat until all of the scrub is used. Rinse off with warm, then cool, water.

Yield: approximately 8 ounces, 1 treatment

Yogurt Body Treatment

*Y*ogurt is one of my favorite beauty treats. It can be used to condition, cleanse, and moisturize your skin and hair, and is rich in vitamins, protein, and calcium. If your skin seems dull or colorless, use this treatment to make it glow. If you have oily skin, omit the oil in this recipe.

2 cups plain yogurt
1 tablespoon wheat germ
1 tablespoon light oil, such as
   apricot kernel or almond oil
1 tablespoon honey

Mix together all ingredients.

To use: Slather all over the body, including the hair, and massage well. Rinse the body in a warm shower followed by a cool rinse—as cold as you can stand it.

Yield: 16 ounces, 1 treatment

DRY BRUSHING

Dry brushing is a popular spa treatment that you can easily do yourself at home before bathing. This treatment opens up clogged pores by removing dead skin cells and surface debris. The boost it gives your skin's circulation is also believed to eliminate cellulite.

Dry brushing is simple and takes about 5 to 10 minutes. You should try it head to toe before bathing. You will want to start out gently and, once your skin is used to this type of treatment, work your way up to more vigorous brushing. Note: Never use dry brushing on your face, and women should avoid the breast area.

To try this treatment you will need a soft, natural-fiber body brush the size of your palm. Dry brushing is done on dry skin—do not use lotion, oils, or water on your skin or the brush. Just begin brushing your hands first, followed by the arms, neck, chest, stomach, and back. Brush in smooth, flowing strokes and do not apply too much pressure. This treatment should feel pleasurable, not painful. Now go on to each leg, starting at the foot. When you are finished, you will feel invigorated and your skin will be glowing.

Following dry brushing you should shower or bathe as you usually do, washing away all the dead skin cells you just exfoliated from your body. Your skin will feel incredibly clean and soft. You should also feel healthier. Many people believe dry brushing removes toxins from their entire system. When you step from the bath, do not rub your skin dry, pat it with a warm fluffy towel and apply a light skin oil or moisturizer.

Keep your dry brush clean by washing it in a mild soap once a week and allowing it to air-dry completely.

English Ivy Body Massage

For years ivy has been used by women as a cure for cellulite because it stimulates circulation and helps rid the body of excess fluids. This lovely green massage cream is a wonderful treat before a shower, and a great way to start the day. It's especially effective when combined with steam from the bath or shower. English ivy is a very popular plant and is found in many gardens and yards. Make sure the leaves you pick are fresh and clean and have not been treated with any pesticides. Remember: Ivy is not an edible plant.

20 fresh English ivy leaves
1 cup distilled water
¼ teaspoon powdered borax
¼ cup almond oil
1½ teaspoons grated beeswax

In a blender or food processor, blend together the ivy leaves and distilled water on high speed for 1 minute. Strain this green ivy water into a clean jar and discard what you have strained off (small bits of leaves).

Measure ½ cup ivy water and mix with the powdered borax. Set aside.

Mix together in an ovenproof glass container the almond oil and beeswax. Gently heat the oil-wax mixture until the wax has melted. You can do this by microwaving for 1 to 2 minutes on High, watching carefully, or by placing the oil-wax container in a pan with 2 inches of water and heating gently over medium heat on the stove top.

When the wax has melted, heat the ivy water mixture, but do not boil. Use the microwave for 1 minute on High, or place the ivy mixture in the same water bath you used to melt the wax. Now, slowly pour the ivy mixture into the oil mixture.

Pour the entire mixture into a blender and blend on high speed for 1 to 2 minutes, or stir vigorously with a small whisk. Pour the mixture into a clean container and allow to cool completely. You will have a lovely thick, green cream.

To use: Before showering, take a small amount of the ivy massage cream in your hand and massage well into your body. Give special attention to your legs, hips, and buttocks. In the shower, using a clean cotton washcloth, scrub your whole body with warm water. Before leaving the shower, rinse your body with the coldest water you can stand.

Yield: 4 ounces

Green Goddess Body Mask

It is important to eat plenty of fresh fruits and vegetables, which help to produce healthy skin and hair from the inside out. Fresh "green" ingredients are also something to put on your body. These ingredients come from the vegetable bin and smell a bit like a freshly tossed salad as they add moisture to your skin, making it feel soft and smooth.

1 cup sliced fresh carrot root
2 cups fresh spinach leaves
½ cup sliced mushrooms
2 cups fresh, sliced zucchini squash
½ cup vegetable water (see
   instructions) or fresh water
½ cup French green clay or any
   natural clay

Combine all the fresh vegetables in a steamer or microwave-safe container. Steam until they are soft and tender and can easily be pierced with a fork. Let the vegetables cool completely and save ½ cup of their cooking water as the vegetable water. Place the cooked vegetables and water in a blender or food processor and process until smooth. Using a fork or whisk, stir in the natural clay. When you finish mixing you should have a smooth, pale green, creamy mixture.

To use: Spread the mask all over your body using your fingers or a small paintbrush. Let the mixture sit on your skin for 10 to 15 minutes. Wrap an old towel around yourself and lie down if you like. Rinse off the body mask in a warm shower and use a rich moisturizer afterward.

Yield: 10 ounces, enough for 1 treatment

Loofah Body Polish

¼ cup ground sea salt or kosher salt
1 loofah sponge

To enhance the effectiveness of your loofah sponge, try this body scrub recipe. It will help keep your skin healthy and glowing by removing any dead, flaky skin and boosting your circulation. Please note that this treatment is intended for your body only; the scrub is too harsh for delicate facial skin.

In the bath or shower, pat the sea salt onto damp skin and gently run the loofah sponge over your skin in a circular pattern. Pay particular attention to classic rough skin spots such as elbows, knees, and heels. Rinse well and follow with a rich body lotion.

Yield: 2 ounces, enough for 1 whole-body treatment

Mehndi— Henna Tattoos

¼ cup boiling water
2 tea bags (orange pekoe or black tea works best)
¼ cup henna powder, finely sifted (Make sure to remove large stems and leaves.)
fresh lemon juice

If you are looking for a new type of body adornment you may want to try a henna tattoo or Mehndi. This ancient art of decorating the body with elaborate henna designs has become popular with everyone from teens to Hollywood stars. Many salons now offer henna tattoos to their customers.

The ancient practice of dying the skin with henna comes from India where the young bride's hands and feet are decorated before her wedding. As the henna is gently painted onto the young girl, family members impart words of wisdom to her. Designs are drawn on top of the skin using a paste made from crushed henna leaves and tea. Though it is temporary, it may last for several weeks.

Pour the boiling water over the tea bags to make a strong tea. Let steep for at least an hour. Place your sifted henna in a glass or ceramic bowl. Slowly add the tea until you have a smooth creamy paste (you may not use all of the tea). Let the mixture sit for several hours, or even overnight, to let the color come out of the henna. If the mixture seems too dry, add a bit more water or tea and stir well. The paste should look like toothpaste in consistency. Decide on your design and where you want it to go. Make sure your skin is clean. Natural oils and lotions can prevent the henna from working. I would start with a simple, small design.

To paint with your henna paste: Place it in a pastry bag or plastic bag with one corner snipped off, or use a small brush. What you use for application will depend on your design. Write with the henna wherever you wish the design to appear. It will stain, so be careful. Once you have finished your design, let the henna dry on your skin, dabbing it every now and then with a slice of lemon. The skin absorbs the henna dye slowly, so keeping it moist will help; the longer it sits on your skin the darker the design will be. Some people cover their designs and leave the henna on overnight. I have let mine sit for 2 to 3 hours and was satisfied with the color. Rinse off the henna with warm water and rub the design with more lemon juice. Voila! Your design will darken a bit more as the lemon juice dries. Mehndi should last for several weeks to a month, depending upon where you made your design on your body and how often it is washed.

Yield: 2 ounces

SUN SENSE

Spending a day outdoors under the warm sun is one of life's greatest treats. The sun is a wonderful source of vitamin D, which is essential for strong bones. However, when you are outdoors, the following guidelines will help protect your skin and hair.

- Always use sun protection. Use a good commercial sunscreen with an SPF rating of 15 or higher. It is difficult to create at-home sunscreens with the proper skin protection.

- Avoid being out in direct sunlight during the middle of the day. This is usually between the hours of 10:00 A.M. and 2:00 P.M. when the sun is strongest.

- Always wear sunglasses. Sunglasses are one of your best beauty tools for slowing down wrinkling around the eyes, and they help to protect your eyes from harmful sunrays.

- Cover your hair with a scarf or hat if out in the direct sunlight for a long period of time, as the sun can be very drying. This is especially important if you dye your hair, because the sun can also lighten the color. You can also spread a small amount of sunscreen on your hair for protection.

If you are unlucky enough to have gotten sunburned, these treatments can help take some of the heat out of the burn. I speak from experience—on many a family vacation I've earned the nickname "the lobster." Remember to keep your skin well moisturized and drink plenty of liquids; sunburn can be very dehydrating to the body.

Apply your sunburn soother in one of the following three methods:

1. Using thin fabric that will cling when wet, such as cheesecloth, silk, or cotton, dip the cloth in the liquid and wrap around your sunburned body. You may have to repeat as the fabric dries. Remember to use a good lotion after these cures, as they can be drying to the skin.

2. Add 1 to 2 cups of sunburn soother to your bathwater. Make sure the water is tepid, not hot. Moisturize your skin well after your bath to replace lost moisture.

3. Apply sunburn soother directly on the skin with a spray bottle. Do not rub the solution into the skin. Let dry and repeat if necessary after the solution has dried. Moisturize your skin well with a rich body lotion.

Yield: 8 to 16 ounces, enough for 1 treatment

Sunburn Soothers

1 to 2 cups of one of the products from the following list of soothers (You may want to dilute some of them with an equal amount of water if you have sensitive skin.)
Witch hazel
Apple cider vinegar (mix with water, 1 tablespoon per cup of water)
Cucumber juice
White wine
Gin
Buttermilk
Cornstarch
Baking soda

Massage Oils and Aromatherapy

*I*f you have ever been given a massage, you know what a wonderful feeling it can bring! It can relax you and relieve tension, and energy is restored to your body as blood flow is stimulated. Oils and lotions are often used by masseurs to enhance the experience. The scents from these oils can create certain moods or mental states — the scent of peppermint, for example, can be very energizing.

Aromatherapy works through our sense of smell, which affects how we eat, our sexual drive, and our behavior in general. It is not a new practice, but is, in fact, very ancient, dating back some five thousand years. Ancient Egyptians perfected the practice and used incense, perfume, and essential oils in medicine, cosmetics, and massage either to heal or to create certain moods. The Babylonians, Greeks, and Romans also used scents and aromatic ingredients. In the early 1900s, René-Maurice Gattefossé, a French chemist, coined the term *aromathérapie*.

Massage oils and aromatherapy are both very effective in changing the physical and mental states of individuals. One of the best gifts my husband can give me after an especially hectic day is a relaxing massage. The recipes in this chapter provide a sampling of scented massage oils that can make the experience even better. Once you have mastered the basic techniques, try to create your own! Massages and oils also make very personal and appreciated gifts.

The products contained in this chapter require the general care and storage guidelines found on page 8. Shelf life for these products is long, with some oils lasting for up to two years.

HOW TO GIVE A GREAT MASSAGE

1. First, choose a massage oil or lotion recipe or simply use a favorite light oil, such as sunflower, almond, or sesame. You may add a drop or two of a selected essential oil to your oil or lotion for a bit of aromatherapy.

2. Locate a place for your massage. Choose a firm, steady surface. Beds are really not such a good location since soft mattresses absorb most of the impact of your massage strokes, stealing the benefits from your body. A massage table is ideal, but you can also use a futon, yoga mat, or layers of quilts and blankets on the floor. Make sure the environment is relaxing—no bright lights overhead or loud noises. Soft music is a nice option.

3. Massage is a physical activity for the giver as well as the recipient. Keep your strokes smooth and flowing. Avoid any sudden moves or interruptions. Keep your stroking toward the heart, not away from it. Your veins have little valves in them that keep the blood flowing toward the heart; you can cause damage to them if you are pushing them in the opposite direction.

4. Take your directions from your partner for areas that feel good or need special attention. Massage is like any other relationship in that it requires communication.

5. After the massage, linger and relax. Listen to a favorite song, read a book, or share a relaxing beverage. Savor the moment.

Amorous Massage Oil

This lightly scented, spicy oil makes a wonderful gift for a couple who deserve a special treat, or for anyone you love. Poured into a red glass bottle with a big bow, it makes a perfect valentine! (Conveniently, the scent of cinnamon is believed to be an aphrodisiac.) Other romantic scents to try are musk, sandalwood, and rose. I have found that men particularly enjoy the scent of this oil.

½ cup light oil (I use canola oil but any light unscented oil will do.)
½ teaspoon ground cinnamon
½ teaspoon vanilla extract

Mix all the ingredients together.

Let the mixture sit for several hours to allow the oil to absorb the cinnamon and vanilla. Pour mixture into a clean jar or bottle through a funnel lined with a coffee filter to remove any solids in the oil. Cover your container and enjoy!

Note: This oil—like all of the scented massage oils— makes a nice body oil to use after a bath or shower. You may also want to try a little nutmeg in addition to the cinnamon in this oil.

Yield: approximately 4 ounces

Herb Massage Oil

½ cup of your favorite light oil (almond, canola, olive, etc.)
1 tablespoon fresh herb or a combination of herbs (See the list at right below for suggested herbs and the moods they can create.)

Herbs are perfect for making scented massage oils because of their strong scents. This recipe can also be used while bathing—pour a tablespoon or two into the bath, as you would scented bath oils. With fresh herbs, I like to save an extra sprig or two to place inside the bottle.

Mix together the oil and the herb or herbs.

Heat gently in the microwave or on the stove top, but do not boil. (I usually microwave on High for 2 minutes.)

Cool the oil mixture completely, about 30 minutes. Filter out all of the solids in the oil by pouring through a funnel filled with a coffee filter into a clean glass jar or bottle. Use and enjoy.

Stimulating herbs

Rosemary	Cures apathy and is good for the memory
Oregano	Boosts circulation
Mint	Energizing; raises your metabolism

Relaxing herbs

Chamomile	Relaxing; cures insomnia
Lavender	Soothing, calming; cures headaches
Basil	Calms the nerves, cures stress; good for decision making, helps concentration

Yield: 4 ounces

Citrus Massage Oil

I grew up around citrus orchards. My father and both of my grandfathers were orange growers in southern California. This is why many of my recipes contain oranges, lemons, grapefruits, limes, and tangerines. You can use any combination of citrus zest in this recipe to create exciting and uplifting oils.

½ cup assorted citrus zest (the colored part of the peel)
½ cup light oil (I like to use almond oil.)

Place the zest in a glass or ceramic bowl. Pour the oil over the zest and heat in the microwave until warm (about 2 minutes on High). If you do not have a microwave, the oil can be heated separately on the stove top and poured over the citrus zest.

Cool completely to allow all of the essential oils from the zest to be released, about 30 minutes. Remove all of the zest from the oil, using a slotted spoon. Pour the oil into a clean jar or bottle.

Note: You can also use this oil when making hand or body creams and lotions.

Yield: 4 ounces

Sore Muscle Massage Oil

½ cup light vegetable oil
½ teaspoon camphor oil

*C*amphor is soothing to tired and sore muscles because it has a cooling effect on the skin. After a tough workout or a big move, this oil, together with a good massage, is a welcome gift. I have found that eucalyptus oil works equally well as a muscle soother. Both these oils can be found at the drugstore.

Combine the oils and pour into a clean bottle.

Yield: 4 ounces

Oil of Oils

2 tablespoons peanut oil
2 tablespoons avocado oil
2 tablespoons sesame oil
2 tablespoons almond oil

Other oils to try:
apricot kernel, canola, coconut, corn, hazelnut, peach kernel, safflower, sunflower, walnut, wheat germ

I like to think that this oil combines the best of all my favorite oils. If you are feeling adventurous or have a collection of different oils in the cupboard, mix up your own unique "oil of oils"! This recipe is perfect for massages or after bathing. You can also add a teaspoon of a favorite scent or a few drops of essential oil to this recipe.

Combine all the oils in a bottle and shake well.

Yield: 4 ounces

Gardenia Oil

*I*n my yard I have a gardenia bush that I love. I hate to throw out the flowers after they have withered, so I now make them into a lovely floral oil that preserves their sweet scent. You can use any fragrant flower petals in this recipe, such as rose, magnolia, lavender, jasmine, or lilac. This oil is best if allowed to sit for at least one week before using.

1 to 2 cups gardenia petals, or your choice of flower petals
2 cups light vegetable oil (I like to use apricot kernel or light olive oil.)

Place the flower petals in a large ceramic container with a lid. Pour the oil over the flower petals. Place the container with the petals and oil in a cool, dark place for at least one week.

Strain off the flower petals, and pour the oil into a clean bottle with a tight-fitting lid or cork. For a stronger scent, you may repeat the process, using the scented oil and more fresh flower petals.

Use this oil for massages and after your bath or shower.

Note: You can also use this oil when making hand and body creams.

Yield: 16 ounces

Cooling Massage Spirits

Some people prefer to use alcohol for massages. It can be especially refreshing in hot climates and during the summer months. The glycerine and castor oil in this recipe will help to keep your skin well moisturized, but you still need to follow up with a good allover body lotion, as the alcohol can be drying to your skin.

2 cups vodka or witch hazel
2 teaspoons glycerine or light corn
  syrup
½ teaspoon castor oil
2–3 drops favorite scent (optional)

Mix together all ingredients and shake or stir well. Pour into a clean container with a tight-fitting lid.

Use to massage the body in place of massage oils.

Yield: 16 ounces

Zanzibar Foot Oil

Off the east coast of Africa in the Indian Ocean lies Zanzibar. The island is famous for its lush and very fragrant spice plantations, where cloves, cinnamon, and pepper are abundant. (Seventy-five percent of the world's cloves comes from Zanzibar.) This massage oil is especially well suited for foot massages because it contains clove oil, which is naturally antiseptic. Clove oil is available at many pharmacies, or you can make your own by soaking a few whole cloves in a tablespoon of oil overnight.

¼ cup light sesame oil or macadamia
  nut oil
⅛ teaspoon clove oil

Mix together the two oils and pour into a clean container.

To use: Massage a small amount into tired feet and legs.

Yield: 2 ounces

Vintage Oil

*G*rape seed oil is the most common carrier oil for commercial massage oils because it is light and hypoallergenic. It is expressed from grape seeds and is easy to find at any natural food store. In France, the first "vinotherapy" spa just opened where grape seed oil massages are offered to clients followed by a warm bubble bath and a glass of wine. Create your own spa experience at home without the jet lag.

½ cup grape seed oil
½ teaspoon dried orange zest
½ teaspoon dried lavender
1 small cinnamon stick
2 whole clove buds

Place all ingredients in a clean, dry bottle and cap tightly with a cork or lid. Shake gently and let sit for 1 to 2 weeks. You may strain the oil through paper coffee filters if you like. I often leave it unstrained, as I like the look of the dried ingredients floating in my oil.

To use: Pour a small amount into your hands and massage into your skin.

Yield: 4 ounces

NATURAL ENERGY

Fatigue or lack of energy is a common complaint today. We are all trying to pack a lot of living into our 24-hour day, and more energy is something we all desire. The key to boosting your energy is not a huge secret, in fact—your mother was right—a healthy diet, plenty of exercise, and a good night's sleep will do more for your energy level than anything else. Here are a few more tips to follow:

- **H_2O:** Make water your drink of choice. Water is crucial for keeping your body running smoothly and your mind sharp. Dehydration is often confused with fatigue so drink at least 8 glasses of water each day.

- **Color:** Use color in your life to create an energy field around your body. Color is visible light energy; choose bright uplifting hues such as red, orange, or yellow to motivate and lift your spirits.

- **Scent:** Aromatherapy really works to refresh your body and mind. Choose energizing scents such as bergamot, eucalyptus, geranium, rosemary, peppermint, and lemon. Add a few drops of essential oil to your cosmetic products and recipes.

- **Breathe:** One of the easiest methods for increasing your energy level is something we all do every day—breathe. Learn to breathe deeply; with each breath feel your body become refocused and reenergized.

- **Sleep:** If you want to look and feel younger and have more energy—get more sleep! Go to bed and wake up at the same time each day (including weekends). Maintaining a consistent sleep cycle will help you sleep more soundly and wake up refreshed.

Hair-Care Products

Great-looking hair is something everyone desires, and it is not difficult to achieve. If you eat well-balanced meals, drink plenty of water, and get plenty of rest, it will be reflected in your skin and hair. Proper hair care and conditioning is vital. The most important thing you can do for your hair is to keep it clean and well nourished.

Hair-care products such as shampoos, conditioners, rinses, and styling aids all perform specific functions that keep your hair looking and feeling its best. Shampoo is intended to clean the scalp first, and hair second, by loosening dirt and oils. Conditioners protect the hair from drying out and becoming too brittle, which can result in breakage. Rinses clean the hair thoroughly and help to remove any other hair-product traces. Styling aids help add body to limp hair, and keep your style in place.

The products contained in this chapter require the general care and storage guidelines found on page 8.

SHAMPOO TIPS

Shampoo is liquid soap for washing your hair, a combination of water, detergent, and some type of fat or oil. How often or where you wash your hair is a matter of personal choice, but keeping it clean is important. Here are a few guidelines I use when washing my hair:

- Use a small amount of shampoo (the size of a quarter); it is better to repeat the amount than waste too much the first time.

- Pour the shampoo into the palm of your hand, never directly onto your head. Rub your palms together gently to create a lather before applying the shampoo to your hair.

- Remember to massage the shampoo into your scalp to get it really clean. A clean scalp is important for healthy hair.

- Rinse well for at least two full minutes and use the coolest water you can stand. My mother always told me that the colder the water, the greater the shine!

- Dry your hair gently; blot rather than rub dry with a towel. I like to make a turban-style hat out of my bath towel and wear it on my head for ten to twenty minutes. This helps absorb the water.

- Always use a wide-toothed comb on wet hair, never a brush.

Most people prefer their shampoo in liquid or cream form. Extra ingredients are often added to shampoos for desired treatments or benefits, such as more body or shine. The following two recipes are for basic shampoos. The first one will seem thinner in consistency than most commercial shampoos. I assure you that the results are equivalent.

Basic Shampoo A

Mix together all the ingredients. Pour the shampoo into a clean squeeze bottle or empty shampoo bottle.

Shampoo as you would normally and rinse well with cool water.

Yield: 4 ounces

¼ cup water
¼ cup liquid soap, such as castile or one for sensitive skin
½ teaspoon light vegetable oil (If you have very oily hair you may want to omit the oil.)

Basic Shampoo B

Mix together all the ingredients. Pour the shampoo into a clean squeeze bottle or empty shampoo bottle. Let the mixture sit overnight to thicken.

Shampoo as you would normally and rinse well with cool water.

Yield: 16 ounces

1 cup water
½ cup liquid soap or inexpensive shampoo
½ cup glycerine
¼ cup borax powder

Herbal Shampoo

½ cup water
2 tablespoons dried or ⅓ cup fresh
    chamomile, lavender, or rosemary
½ cup Basic Shampoo (see page 173)
    or mild commercial shampoo
2 tablespoons glycerine

*C*ertain herbs added to your favorite shampoo can bring out your hair's natural highlights. Chamomile makes a mild shampoo that is perfect for fine, light-colored hair; the flowers have a mild bleaching effect. If you have dark-colored hair, I would suggest using rosemary or lavender to enhance your own natural color.

Mix together the water and herbs and heat gently to make a strong tea. Let the mixture steep for at least 20 minutes. Add the shampoo and glycerine to the herbal water mixture and stir well.

Pour the shampoo into a clean squeeze bottle or empty shampoo bottle. Let the mixture sit overnight to thicken.

Shampoo as you would normally and rinse well.

Yield: 8 ounces

Egg Shampoo

1 raw egg
1 tablespoon Basic Shampoo
    (see page 173) or your favorite
    shampoo

*F*or years I have used a raw egg on my hair to give it extra body and shine. Simply apply a raw egg to your hair and massage it into your scalp and hair as you would shampoo. Use cool to warm water when rinsing it out. (Very hot water will leave you with scrambled eggs in your hair; this is not fun to pick out!) This recipe is a simple variation on the basic egg shampoo but is just as effective. If you are not going to use the shampoo immediately, you will need to refrigerate this mixture, as raw eggs spoil easily.

Mix together the raw egg and the shampoo.

Shampoo your hair as you would normally, using cool water (as cool as you can stand). Rinse well for at least 1 minute.

Yield: 1 ounce, 1 application

Body and Bounce Beer Shampoo

Beer is one of my favorite beauty treatments for hair—nothing else gives my hair such body, bounce, and shine. This shampoo is a cinch to make and really works. After you've tried it, you'll never again throw out flat or stale beer.

1 cup beer (Any inexpensive beer will do—fresh or flat.)
1 cup Basic Shampoo (see page 173) or inexpensive commercial shampoo

Heat the beer in a small saucepan over medium heat and boil until the beer is reduced to ¼ cup. Add the reduced beer to the shampoo and stir well.

Pour the shampoo into a clean squeeze bottle or empty shampoo bottle. (You do not need to refrigerate this product.)

Shampoo as you would normally and rinse well.

Yield: 10 ounces

Desert Wonder Shampoo

The aloe vera plant is sometimes called "the wonder of the desert" because of its many uses, especially as a moisturizer for dry skin and hair. Desert conditions can be extremely hard on the hair and this shampoo helps replace lost moisture and oils. I leave it in my hair for a few extra minutes to allow the aloe and oil to soak in.

¼ cup Basic Shampoo (see page 173) or liquid soap
¼ cup aloe vera gel
1 teaspoon glycerine
½ teaspoon avocado oil

Mix together all the ingredients.

Pour into a clean shampoo container with a tight-fitting lid. Shampoo as you would normally, then let it remain on the hair for a few extra minutes. Rinse well with cool water.

Note: This shampoo may separate; always shake well to remix before using.

Yield: 4 ounces

Sunshine Shampoo

¼ cup Basic Shampoo (see page 173)
  or liquid soap
2 tablespoons fresh lemon juice
¼ cup water
½ teaspoon dried citrus peel or
  1 tablespoon fresh citrus zest
  (the colored part of the peel,
  removed with a sharp knife or
  zester)

Citrus scents are clean and fresh and make you feel energized, as if you've spent a day in the sun! This recipe contains fresh lemon juice, which can have a mild bleaching effect on the hair. If you have light-colored hair, it is the perfect shampoo to use during the summer months when your hair is highlighted by the sun. This recipe is also good for oily hair.

Mix together all ingredients. Heat the mixture gently; do not boil. (I put the mixture in the microwave on High for 1 to 2 minutes.)

Cool the mixture completely and strain out the citrus zest. Pour the citrus shampoo into a clean bottle with a tight-fitting lid.

Shampoo as you normally would and rinse well with cool water.

Yield: 4 ounces

Olive Oil Shampoo

½ cup water
¼ cup olive oil
1 cup liquid soap or mild shampoo

Olive oil conditions and improves the strength of your hair. You can add your favorite fragrance to this shampoo as you're blending the ingredients. If your hair is a little oily, cut back on the amount of olive oil.

Blend together all ingredients until smooth.

Pour the shampoo into a clean bottle with a tight-fitting lid. Shampoo as you would normally and rinse well with cool water.

Note: You may need to shake this shampoo before using to remix the ingredients.

Yield: 12 ounces

Dry Shampoos

Using a dry shampoo can be an effective way to remove grease and dirt from your hair without getting it wet. Some people like to use dry shampoos when they are camping and water supplies are scarce. Using a dry shampoo can be a bit messy, so make sure you stand on a towel or lean over a sink while shampooing. I have found that dry shampoos leave my hair clean and shiny, but with a little static electricity. To avoid this, use a natural-bristle brush afterward. You may also want to place a piece of gauze over your brush to absorb dirt and oil. These shampoos can be used to clean wigs and hairpieces.

1 tablespoon dry shampoo powder
(see list at left below)

Dry shampoos to try:

Salt: Make sure you use coarse or kosher salt, as regular cooking salt is too fine and you'll have trouble getting it all out.

Cornmeal: This leaves the hair really shiny. It is the most popular dry shampoo.

Semolina flour: This is the coarse flour used in making pasta and is similar to cornmeal in results.

Orrisroot powder: Leaves the hair with a mild violet scent. This is a finer powder and takes a little extra brushing to remove.

Massage the powder directly into the scalp and through the hair. You may want to lean over a sink as you apply the powder. Leave it on for at least 15 minutes.

Using a clean, dry brush, vigorously brush, using upward strokes, to remove all of the powder. Make sure you are outside, over a sink, or standing on a towel, as this can be messy.

Yield: 1 ounce, 1 dry shampoo

Basil Shampoo Powder

Basil gives the hair luster and shine. This shampoo powder is especially convenient when traveling or backpacking because it is so light and compact. For extra highlighting, blondes may want to add a little chamomile to this powder, and brunettes can add rosemary or lavender.

½ cup finely grated castile soap (see page 255, or use a commercial product)
2 teaspoons borax powder
1 teaspoon baking soda
1 tablespoon dried basil leaves or 3 tablespoons fresh basil leaves, chopped fine

Mix together all ingredients. Store in an airtight container. (I use a resealable plastic bag.)

To use: Pour a small amount into your palm and add a little water to form a paste. Massage into your scalp and through your hair. Rinse well and follow with a good conditioner.

Yield: 4 ounces

Rice Flour Dry Shampoo

This is a recipe that contains a combination of two popular dry shampoos, rice flour and baking soda. Cornstarch could also be used in place of the rice flour.

½ cup rice flour
1 teaspoon baking soda
1 tablespoon borax powder

Mix together all ingredients. Massage the powder directly into the scalp and through the hair. You may want to lean over a sink as you apply the powder.

Leave the powder on for at least fifteen minutes. Using a clean, dry brush, vigorously brush out all of the powder. Make sure you are outside, over a sink, or standing on a towel, as this can be messy.

Yield: 5 ounces

CONDITIONING HAIR PACKS

I once visited a new hair salon in Portland, Oregon. The stylist was amazed at how healthy my hair was—she could not believe that I used electric rollers and a blow-dryer on my hair every day. I told her that I used a once-a-week hair pack of mayonnaise. Another client asked if it was one of the latest cholesterol treatments being sold at the salon. "No," I replied, "just normal mayonnaise from the grocery store." That night I am sure the stylist and several of the other customers were wearing mayonnaise hair packs on their heads. Homemade beauty treatments are contagious!

Conditioning hair packs are rich in natural creams and oils. They are massaged into your hair and left on to allow the rich ingredients to penetrate. They are especially effective for dry hair and hair that has been damaged by too much sun or blow-drying. A weekly hair pack after shampooing will return moisture and life to your hair.

To make your own natural hair packs, choose one or a combination of the products from the following list, for example, avocado and mayonnaise. Use approximately ¼ cup, less or more depending on your hair length. Apply the mixture to clean, damp hair. Wrap your hair with a large piece of plastic wrap or use a plastic shower cap to hold in heat and open up the hair follicles for deep conditioning.

(continued)

Wait 15 minutes and rinse thoroughly with cool water.

Conditioning packs to try:

For dry hair: coconut oil, banana, avocado, mayonnaise

For normal hair: mayonnaise, egg, olive oil, plain yogurt

For oily hair: Add a little lemon juice (1 to 2 teaspoons) to the products for normal hair.

Honey (Molasses) Hair Pack

½ cup honey or molasses (You may need to use a little more if you have very long hair.)

Honey can do great things for hair that has been mistreated and damaged by giving it back color, moisture, body, and shine. It will also lighten your hair slightly, so for dark-haired individuals I would suggest using molasses. This treatment is a little sticky, but well worth it. Don't worry—it rinses out of your hair very easily.

Massage the honey into your hair and leave on for 20 to 30 minutes. You may cover your head with a plastic shower cap or plastic wrap.

Wash and condition your hair as you do normally.

Yield: 4 ounces, 1 hair pack

Perfect Hair Conditioner

My sister Mariann has beautiful dark brown hair with wonderful texture and body. Recently, she moved with her husband to Chicago—the windy city!—where weather conditions are hard on the skin and hair. She uses this conditioner once a week to keep her hair soft, radiant, and the envy of all her friends.

1 teaspoon almond oil
1 teaspoon avocado oil
1 teaspoon olive oil
1 egg yolk
1 tablespoon honey
1 tablespoon fresh lemon juice

Mix all the ingredients together and stir thoroughly.

Massage into your hair and scalp. Wrap your hair in plastic wrap or use a plastic shower cap and leave the conditioner on your hair for 15 minutes.

Shampoo your hair as usual and rinse well.

Yield: approximately 2 ounces, enough for 1 treatment

Rock Melon Hair Conditioner

Rock melon is another name for cantaloupe, an apt one if you've ever seen them growing in a garden; these round fruits do resemble a round rock. Rock melon makes a wonderful light conditioner, especially if you have oily hair, as it is not full of extra creams and oils.

½ cup mashed cantaloupe (Use a fork to create a smooth consistency—it is all right if it seems a bit watery.)

Massage the cantaloupe into your hair before or after you have shampooed. Leave the cantaloupe in your hair for 10 minutes.

Rinse well with warm to cool water.

Yield: 1 treatment

Roaring Twenties Conditioner

1 packet unflavored gelatin, about
   1 tablespoon
¼ cup warm water
1 egg
2 tablespoons fresh lemon juice

When my grandmother was a young girl in the twenties, automobiles were still open and she and her friends would wrap huge chiffon scarves around their heads to protect their hair from the wind. Once a week she would also use an egg conditioner in her hair. The protein and lecithin contained in eggs keep the hair soft and smooth. This recipe is based on a hair conditioner she remembers using.

Dissolve the gelatin in the warm water, stirring well. Add the egg and lemon juice to the gelatin mixture.

Shampoo your hair as usual. Rub the conditioner into your hair and leave on for 1 to 2 minutes.

Rinse thoroughly with warm water (rinse for at least 1 minute), then finish with a cool-water rinse.

Yield: 3 ounces, enough for 1 application

Tucson Jojoba Oil and Beer Conditioner

1 cup warm beer
1 teaspoon jojoba oil

Tucson is a city in southern Arizona, close to the Mexican border. Jojoba plants grow wild here in the desert and you can purchase the oil at many local markets. Native Americans and Mexicans use this oil as a hair and skin conditioner. It is very light and nongreasy—it will solidify like coconut oil if it gets too cold. I like to use local Mexican beers in this recipe, but any inexpensive brand will do.

Mix together the beer and jojoba oil. Make sure the beer is warm or the oil will turn hard (chemically, jojoba oil is similar to wax).

To use: Pour the conditioner over your head and massage into your scalp and through your hair. Rinse well. You may want to lightly shampoo and rinse again, using straight beer if your hair feels a bit too oily.

Yield: 1 treatment

Caribbean Rum Conditioner

*T*wo years ago my whole family took a cruise through the Caribbean islands. In Puerto Rico we toured a famous rum factory, where the popular liquor is made primarily with molasses. I knew how beneficial honey and molasses were to dry, damaged hair, so I was inspired to use this rum in creating a new hair treatment. After using it my hair had more body and shine and was really soft.

3 tablespoons rum
1 egg

Mix the rum and egg together and stir well.

After shampooing, pour the mixture into your hair and leave it in for 1 to 2 minutes. Rinse well with the coolest water you can stand. (Water that is too hot may leave you with scrambled eggs in your hair!)

Yield: 3 ounces, enough for 1 application

Dandruff-Control Treatments

*D*andruff is the most common of all scalp problems, characterized by dry, flaky skin on or about the hair roots. The causes of dandruff are many—lack of proper hair care, poor diet, stress, fatigue, climate, and heredity are all factors. For serious cases of scalp dryness, you should consult your physician. These two recipes are for a pre-shampoo treatment.

FOR AN OILY, FLAKY SCALP

2 tablespoons apple cider vinegar or
  fresh lemon juice
2 tablespoons distilled water
2 tablespoons olive oil

Mix together all the ingredients and massage into your scalp. Leave on for 20 minutes before shampooing.

Yield: 3 ounces, enough for one treatment

FOR A DRY, FLAKY SCALP

2 tablespoons jojoba oil
¼ teaspoon tea tree oil

Combine the 2 oils and massage into wet hair. Leave on for 10 minutes, then shampoo out.

Yield: 1 ounce, enough for 1 treatment

Natural Hair Rinses

The following is a list of rinses to try after you shampoo and as a final rinse. Remember to always rinse your hair with the coolest water you can stand for at least one full minute after using these rinses. Each recipe makes enough for one application.

LEMON JUICE:

The juice of 1 [3 tbsp] lemon and 1 cup water, mixed, brings back life and shine to dull hair.

BAKING SODA:

1 tablespoon baking soda and 1 cup water, mixed, removes hair spray and gel residue.

APPLE CIDER VINEGAR:

½ cup vinegar and 2 cups water, mixed, gives your hair shine and bounce.

BEER:

1 can or bottle of beer gives body to your hair. Never throw out flat beer—save it for your hair. I have an opened quart of beer in my refrigerator at all times.

TOMATO JUICE:

1 cup of tomato juice will remove any odors, such as smoke, from your hair.

There are also many natural rinses that you can use to color or highlight your hair. These rinses create gradual changes in your hair when used over a period of time; the longer you use them the more dramatic the results. After shampooing try one of the following:

CHAMOMILE:

This will lighten fair hair. To make a rinse, pour 2 cups boiling water over ¼ cup chamomile flowers. Cool; strain before using. 4 tbsp

RHUBARB:

This will also lighten hair. Use ¼ cup chopped, fresh rhubarb to 2 cups boiling water. Cool; strain before using.

SAGE, LAVENDER, AND CINNAMON:

These will darken hair. Use ¼ cup sage or lavender (or 3 cinnamon sticks, broken into small pieces) to 2 cups boiling water. Cool; strain before using.

HIBISCUS FLOWERS:

These will give red highlights to light or dark hair. Use dry flowers or herbal tea containing hibiscus flowers. Steep the flowers in boiling water to the shade you desire. Cool; strain before using. Remember you can always go darker, so start out with a weak mixture.

Watercress Rinse for Oily Hair

1 cup watercress
1 cup water

Watercress sandwiches are a mainstay of many teas and luncheons, but this green also makes an excellent hair rinse. The juice is a mild acid that contains minerals, iron, and phosphorus. It revitalizes oily hair by removing soap residues, thus getting it really clean. Wild watercress can be found growing near streams and springs. You can also purchase it in the produce section of many grocery stores.

Blend together the watercress and water. Strain off any solids and save the liquid.

Pour the watercress rinse on damp, clean hair and leave on for 20 minutes. Rinse well with cool water.

Yield: 8 ounces

Dandruff Rinse

½ cup apple cider vinegar
½ cup fresh or 1 tablespoon dried mint leaves
1 cup boiling water

If you are suffering from a dandruff condition, this rinse may help remove the dry flakes from your hair and scalp. If you have very flaky hair and scalp, and it does not get better, you should see a physician. The vinegar in this rinse is a mild acid that gently clears the scalp of any dead skin cells.

Place the vinegar and mint leaves in a ceramic bowl. Pour the boiling water over the mixture.

Allow the mixture to cool completely, and then strain out the mint leaves.

Apply the remaining solution to the scalp as a final rinse after shampooing. Rinse with cool water as a final step.

Yield: 12 ounces

Henna Hair Color

Henna is a semipermanent hair coloring with a coating action that seals in oils and tightens the hair cuticles to give more shine and luster. One advantage henna offers is that it gradually washes out of your hair while new hair is growing in—this means that you won't develop noticeable roots just a few weeks after dyeing.

When using henna to color your hair, the new color will go through an adjustment period of two to three days. So do not panic if your hair seems brassy or dull—it will probably change.

When choosing a color, remember that hair cannot be made lighter with henna. It can be made darker by leaving the henna on the hair longer, or by choosing a darker shade. I recommend starting out lighter, and reapplying more henna, rather than starting right off with a dark shade. You can also create new colors by mixing together several different hennas, for example, red and brown henna can be used for auburn hair.

One method of testing the final henna color is to do a sample test on your own hair.

Gather up a small sample piece of hair from a place you will not notice—usually near the nape of the neck. Use a rubber band to tightly bind the swatch together.

Mix a small amount of the henna powder with water and dip the hair into it. Wrap the hair in plastic wrap and let it sit for 15 minutes.

Rinse the sample and let dry. Check the hair color in a good strong light; you may even want to go outside.

Once you are satisfied with your henna color choice, follow the directions on the henna powder box. These are the steps I normally use:

½ cup pure henna powder, using your choice of color (You
may need to use more powder if you have very long hair.)
¼ cup boiling water (approximately)

Place the henna powder in a ceramic, glass, or plastic container and slowly add the boiling water, stirring until you have a thick paste the consistency of mud. You may need to add a little more water. *Do not use metal utensils or containers when mixing henna.*

Apply the henna to clean, dry hair. If you are using colored hennas, you may want to wear gloves so as not to stain your hands. Cover your entire head with the henna and massage well into your hair, through to the ends. Wrap your head in plastic wrap or use a plastic shower cap.

Keep your head warm: Sit in the sun, use a handheld blow-dryer and keep it moving, sit under a warm hair dryer, or wrap your head in a warm, wet towel. Do this for 15 to 45 minutes. The longer the henna is left in your hair, the darker the color will become.

Rinse your hair thoroughly with warm water until the water runs clear. Shampoo your hair, using a very mild shampoo, and rinse well. You may now dry and style your hair as usual.

Note: Your henna color should stay in your hair for 3 to 6 months. Henna gradually washes out of your hair.

Yield: 2 to 4 ounces (depending on the length of your hair), 1 treatment

HENNA ENHANCERS

If you've been using henna to condition or color your hair, here are a few new tricks to try. The henna paste I refer to in this section is from the recipe on pages 187–188.

Henna and Egg: To give your hair extra shine, add 1 whole raw egg to your henna paste before putting it on your hair.

Henna and Yogurt: For extra conditioning power, add 2 tablespoons plain yogurt to your henna paste before applying it to your hair. This is especially helpful for dry and brittle hair.

Henna and Spice: For extra highlights and a delicious scent, try adding some spice to your henna paste before applying it to your hair—a small amount (¼ teaspoon) of ginger, nutmeg, allspice, or cinnamon will enrich red and brown hennas and will smell great.

Henna and Vinegar: For golden or copper highlights, add 3 tablespoons apple cider vinegar to your henna paste before applying to your hair.

Henna and Tea: When mixing the henna powder into a paste, use tea instead of water. Use three tea bags for a strong brew. Try black or Ceylon for brunettes, chamomile for blondes, and for black hair use strong black coffee.

Egyptian Henna Conditioning Treatment

½ cup neutral (colorless) pure henna powder (You may need to use more depending on the length of your hair—this amount will cover shoulder-length hair.)

¼ cup boiling water (approximately)

*H*enna was used in ancient Egypt as a dye and conditioner for the hair and nails. Most people think of it as having a reddish brown color; actually, red is only one color henna comes in. My mother uses brown henna to cover her gray hair; there are black and neutral or colorless henna powders as well. If you do not want to change your hair color, I would suggest using only colorless henna. Do not use it if your hair is already colored or has a permanent wave; it could react with these products, which have already been absorbed by your hair.

Note: Most henna powders come with a set of instructions. Always read all instructions carefully before using. The directions for this recipe are the same as those for Henna Hair Color, page 187. Because you are not changing your hair color, there is no need to do the sample test.

Yield: 2 to 4 ounces (depending on hair length), 1 treatment

Basic Hair Gel

1 cup water

1 teaspoon unflavored gelatin (or flavored gelatin of your choice; found in any grocery store)

*F*lavored gelatin can be used to set or style your hair. Gelatin contains sugar and protein, both of which help to repair damaged hair and give it more body. Try some of the many flavors and colors available at the grocery store: blondes can use lemon, redheads raspberry, and brunettes grape!

Heat the water almost to boiling. This can be done in the microwave or on a stove top. Sprinkle the gelatin over the hot water and stir well until the gelatin is completely dissolved. Allow the mixture to cool. (This can be done in the refrigerator.)

When firm to the touch, use a small amount to set and style your hair. You can use this gel on either wet or dry hair to set and style it.

Note: At room temperature, the gel will thin a little. It is just as effective in this state, but if you prefer a thicker hair gel, store in the refrigerator.

Yield: 8 ounces

Pink Grapefruit Styling Gel

Grapefruit juice by itself makes an excellent styling lotion because it is full of natural sugars that help hold the hair in place. The protein from the gelatin in this recipe gives hair extra body. This is a powerful styling gel, strong enough for the most unmanageable hair. I like to comb a small amount through my hair while it is still wet, before I use my blow-dryer. It also works well as a styling gel after drying.

½ cup warm water
1 packet, approximately 1 tablespoon, unflavored gelatin
½ cup fresh pink grapefruit juice
1 teaspoon glycerine
1 crushed vitamin C tablet

Combine the warm water and gelatin. Stir until the gelatin is dissolved. Add the grapefruit juice, glycerine, and vitamin C. Stir the mixture until all ingredients are well mixed.

Refrigerate the mixture until solid (about 2 hours). Remove the solid mixture from the refrigerator. When it warms to room temperature, it will be ready to use. Stir the mixture thoroughly one last time before using.

Store in an airtight container. You can use this gel on either wet or dry hair to set and style it.

Yield: 8 ounces

Almond Oil Hair Gel

1½ cups warm water
1 packet unflavored gelatin,
    approximately 1 tablespoon
1 teaspoon glycerine
1 tablespoon almond oil
¼ teaspoon almond extract (optional,
    for scent)

Heated hairstyling tools, such as curling irons, rollers, and blow-dryers, can be very drying to your hair, especially if used every day. I have added a tablespoon of almond oil to this recipe to help condition the hair and protect it from becoming too dry and brittle.

Combine the warm water and gelatin. Stir until the gelatin is dissolved. Add the glycerine, almond oil, and almond extract, if desired. Stir the mixture until all ingredients are blended well. (Don't worry if the oil floats to the top of the mixture.)

Refrigerate the mixture until it is almost set (about 1 hour). Stir the mixture thoroughly, mixing together the water and the oil. Place back in the refrigerator until set (about another hour).

Remove firm gel from the refrigerator. When it reaches room temperature, it is ready for use. Stir the mixture thoroughly one last time before using.

Store in an airtight container. You can use this gel on either wet or dry hair to set and style it.

Yield: approximately 8 ounces

Champagne Hair Gel

*L*ike beer, champagne (or sparkling wine) is rich in sugar and protein, which help to thicken the hair and give it more bounce. Champagne also works well as a styling lotion. Save a small amount from your next celebration to use in this recipe—don't worry if it has gone flat. This gel can be used on wet or dry hair.

1 packet unflavored gelatin, approximately 1 tablespoon
½ cup warm water
½ cup champagne or sparkling wine
1 tablespoon rose water

Dissolve the gelatin in the warm water and stir well. Add the champagne and rose water and stir well again.

Allow to set into a gel (placing the mixture in the refrigerator will speed up this process). Remove when set, and allow the mixture to reach room temperature before using. Store in an airtight container.

Yield: 8 ounces

Brilliantine

*M*y grandfather always used a brilliantine dressing to hold his hair in place. It contained castor oil, one of the few natural oils soluble in alcohol. Today, brilliantine is still a popular hair oil because it is semi-drying and leaves a tough, shiny film on the hair. Whenever I make this recipe I think of my handsome, well-groomed grandfather.

½ cup vodka
2 tablespoons castor oil

Mix together the vodka and castor oil. Pour into a clean bottle; shake before using.

Comb a small amount through your hair and allow to dry, for extra shine.

Yield: 5 ounces

Rosemary Hair Oil

2 tablespoons dried rosemary
½ cup olive oil

Rosemary is believed to stimulate hair growth. Mixed with olive oil, it makes a hair oil that can be massaged into the scalp. I see this hair oil sold in almost every natural food store I go in, but it's so easy and so much less expensive to make at home.

Mix together the rosemary and olive oil. Heat gently in the microwave or on the stove top, but do not boil. I usually microwave on High for 2 minutes.

Cool the oil mixture completely, and let sit for 2 to 3 days to allow the oil to absorb all of the essential oils from the rosemary.

Filter out all the solids in the oil by pouring through a funnel lined with a coffee filter. Pour into a clean bottle. Use by massaging a small amount into your scalp after shampooing and before going to bed.

Yield: 4 ounces

Jalapeño Hair Tonic

2 small or 1 large jalapeño pepper
½ cup vodka
2 tablespoons castor oil

On a recent trip to Mexico I complimented a beautiful woman working at our hotel on the condition of her hair (it was very thick and shiny), and she shared with me this family recipe. Jalapeño peppers are used to prevent hair loss by stimulating new hair growth. A small amount is rubbed into the scalp by both men and women before retiring in the evening. Make sure you use caution when using peppers, and wash your hands well before touching your face or eyes — the juice can burn.

Chop the jalapeño pepper into tiny pieces and place in a small ceramic bowl. Pour the vodka over the peppers and allow to sit for several days.

Strain off the vodka and discard the peppers. Add the castor oil to the pepper vodka and pour into a clean bottle.

Shake before using. Massage a small amount into your scalp before going to bed (it will cause a slight tingling sensation on your scalp).

Yield: 5 ounces

Lemon Hair Spray

This is an extremely simple hair spray that can be used as either a setting lotion before styling your hair or to hold it in place after styling. The oil from the lemon peel may lighten some hair types, especially if you spend a lot of time in the sun. This recipe works equally well with any citrus peel—tangerine, grapefruit, orange, or a combination.

Zest from 1 lemon peel (yellow part only)
1 cup boiling water
1 tablespoon vodka

Place the lemon zest in a ceramic or glass bowl and pour the boiling water over it. Let sit for several hours or even overnight.

Remove the zest with a slotted spoon. (You can also pour the water through a funnel lined with a coffee filter to remove any solids from the liquid.) Stir the vodka into the lemon-water solution.

Pour this solution into a clean spritzer bottle and use before or after styling your hair. It can be used on both wet and dry hair.

Yield: 8 ounces

Psyllium-Seed Setting Lotion

1 tablespoon psyllium seeds
1 cup hot water
1 tablespoon vodka

*P*syllium seeds are produced by a plant in the plantain family, and are used in hair-setting products because they create a thick gel. This gel surrounds the hair, helping it to hold a set. The seed husks also work in this recipe, but I prefer to use the whole seeds, as they are easier to strain from the liquid. (If you have very dry hair, I would cut down the amount of alcohol or leave it out altogether.)

Soak the psyllium seeds in the hot water for at least 30 minutes. The liquid will become clear and thick. Strain out the seeds and discard. You should have approximately ½ cup of liquid. If you have more, simply measure out ½ cup and either save or discard the rest. Add the vodka to the ½ cup psyllium gel and stir well.

Store in a clean container with a tight-fitting lid. Use this lotion to set your hair.

Yield: 4 ounces

Sugar Hair Spray

1 tablespoon sugar
1 cup warm water

*W*hen my great-grandmother was a girl, she used sugar and water to hold her hair in place and give it extra body. Sugar coats the hair and makes it look thicker. Be careful when using this spray during the summer months, as it may attract bees or mosquitoes.

Dissolve the sugar in the water and stir well to mix. Pour the sugar water into a clean spritzer bottle.

Spray your hair with this spray before setting, or after, to hold your style in place.

Yield: 8 ounces

Swimming Pool Hair Care

Chlorine and chemicals used in many public swimming pools can be harsh and damaging to your hair. When swimming, wear a bathing cap when possible. Wetting your hair with fresh water before you swim will also keep it from soaking up too much chlorine water. Always remember to rinse your hair well after swimming. You may have to bring a bottle of fresh water with you to the pool for just this reason.

Here is a recipe to deep cleanse your hair and remove any built-up chlorine and chemicals. Swimmer's hair can sometimes turn "green" and have a strong chlorine smell. This baking soda treatment will help refresh and restore your hair.

2 tablespoons baking soda
¼ cup fresh lemon juice
1 teaspoon mild shampoo

Mix together all the ingredients until well blended. Wet hair and massage mixture well into hair and scalp, making sure hair ends are coated. Cover hair with a plastic bag or shower cap and leave on for 30 minutes. Rinse hair well and shampoo as usual. Repeat treatment as needed.

Yield: 2 ounces, enough for 1 treatment

Nail Treatments

I have two young children and a household to manage, so it is often easy to forget about proper nail and hand care. My grandmother also worked hard, yet she always made a conscious effort to apply hand cream every time she washed her hands. My mother always carried a nail file in her purse, and has them hidden all over her house—something I now find myself doing.

Healthy and strong nails are really very easy to achieve. Eating a proper diet is essential, as too little protein can make your nails brittle and dull. Keeping them well moisturized is also important, as the nail is extremely porous and gives off moisture a hundred times as fast as the skin. Massaging the cuticle area will increase the circulation and encourage new nail growth. All of these things take minutes to do and the effects are long-lasting.

Always wear gloves when working with cleaning chemicals. I also try to wear gloves when I wash the dishes, while I garden, and at night after I apply cream or oil. Other tips I have collected over the years for strong and flexible nails:

- Keep a bottle or jar of hand cream by all of your sinks.

- Never use your nails as tools. My sister, who has beautiful nails, gave me this tip and it really works.

- Push back your cuticles every time you wash your hands or apply hand cream.

- Never cut your cuticles. The cuticle protects the nail by sealing off the opening between the nail and the skin.

- To keep nails clean while gardening, scratch a bar of soap. Let the soap get under your nails so dirt won't.

- Keep all of your nails the same length.

The products contained in this chapter require the general care and storage guidelines found on page 8.

MANICURE FOR HEALTHY HANDS AND NAILS

Once a week, you should give yourself a manicure—this is essential for healthy nails and soft hands. These same steps can also be followed for the feet and toenails by giving yourself a pedicure.

1. Remove all traces of nail polish, preferably by using a mild nail polish remover and cotton. (I sometimes make my own remover by purchasing some acetone at my drugstore and adding a little glycerine to it.)

2. Soak your nails and fingertips in warm, soapy water for at least 5 minutes. This softens the cuticles and rinses off all the nail polish remover.

3. Apply cuticle cream to the base of your nails. Massage the cream into the cuticles. Gently push back your cuticles with a cotton-tipped stick. (I purchase orange sticks from the drugstore and wrap cotton around the ends.) Never cut your cuticles.

4. File the nails into rounded ovals—never points—and make sure all nails are the same length. Nothing looks worse than four short nails and one long one, or vice versa.

5. Make a hand mask, using your favorite facial mask recipe on your hands. Rinse well with cool water and pat dry. (I like to use the Swiss Milkmaid Mask, page 102.)

6. Massage your entire hand with a rich hand cream or oil. Wrap your hands in plastic wrap or put on cotton gloves and leave on at least 30 minutes or, better, overnight.

7. To polish your nails, rub some light vegetable or mineral oil into them and buff for a natural shine. Buffing also helps increase the circulation and results in healthier nails.

Jojoba Nail and Cuticle Oil

1 teaspoon jojoba oil
1 teaspoon almond oil
½ teaspoon vitamin E oil

One trick for keeping your cuticles soft is to soak your nails in warm water for ten minutes, then rub this oil treatment into the nails and cuticles to lock in the moisture. Jojoba oil is light and nongreasy. It is actually very similar to our own body oils in texture, and is easily absorbed by the skin and nails.

Mix together all three oils. Massage a small amount into your cuticles. (This oil also works well on your feet and toenails.) Store in a clean container.

Yield: 1 ounce

Cocoa Cuticle Cream

2 tablespoons coconut oil
½ teaspoon grated cocoa butter

This is a rich cream that is perfect for massaging into the cuticle at the base of each nail to condition and increase circulation. Massaging this cream daily into your cuticles will keep them soft and help promote healthy nail growth.

Combine coconut oil and coca butter in an ovenproof container and heat gently until melted. Stir well until you have a smooth cream and pour into a clean container. Let the cream cool completely before using.

To use: Massage a small amount into cuticles.

Yield: 1 ounce

Natural Nail Polish

By massaging this mixture into clean nails, you will improve your hand's circulation while promoting new nail growth. The talc or clay enhances the nail's natural luster and works as a gentle polish.

1 tablespoon pure olive oil
½ tablespoon talc or powdered white
   clay

Mix together the olive oil and talc into a smooth cream. If the mixture seems too thick, add a bit more olive oil.

To use: Massage a small amount into your nails and cuticles. Wipe off any excess with a soft cloth or cotton pad and buff lightly for a soft natural glow. Save any extra in a small container with a lid or cover with plastic wrap.

Yield: ½ ounce

Molasses Nail Soak

Pure molasses made from the juice of fresh sugarcane can be used as a soak to soften cuticles and strengthen and condition nails before a manicure. Like honey, molasses is an excellent natural humectant that will help restore lost moisture to the skin and nails. (Don't worry—it won't leave your hands all sticky; it rinses away easily.)

¼ cup warm water
2 tablespoons molasses

Mix together the water and molasses, stirring well.

To use: Soak your nails in the solution for 15 to 20 minutes or swab on clear nails in the evening before going to bed.

Yield: 2 ounces, enough for 1 nail soak for both hands

Pineapple Cuticle Softener

1 egg yolk
2 tablespoons fresh pineapple juice

Pineapple contains an active enzyme called bromelain. It is effective in softening rough, dry skin. It can also be drying, so to counteract this I have added an egg yolk to the recipe.

Mix together the egg yolk and pineapple juice and stir well.

To use: Spread this mixture on your cuticles and let sit for 5 minutes. Using a cotton-covered orange stick or cotton swab, gently push back the softened cuticle skin against your nail bed. Never cut your cuticles as this could damage them. Rinse with warm water to remove the mixture. Then massage some coconut oil or rich hand cream into your hands. Discard any leftover product.

Yield: 1 ounce, enough for 1 treatment

Evening Nail Oil

1 tablespoon olive oil
2 teaspoons liquid lecithin
1 vitamin E capsule, broken open, or
   ¼ teaspoon vitamin E oil

In the evening, as I discuss the day's events with my husband, I like to rub this oil into my nails. It strengthens and conditions them and takes only a few minutes. This is also a good oil to use before buffing your nails — it makes them really shiny!

Combine all ingredients and mix thoroughly. Pour into a clean container. Dab a small amount on your fingers and rub thoroughly into your nails.

Yield: ½ ounce

Nail Hardener

This is a wonderful nail hardener and conditioner. I use a cotton swab and apply the solution to my nails throughout the day and before going to bed at night.

1 tablespoon water
1 tablespoon witch hazel
1½ teaspoons honey
½ teaspoon alum powder

Combine all ingredients and mix thoroughly. Pour into a clean bottle. With a cotton swab, apply the solution to clean, dry nails.

Yield: 1½ ounces

Henna Nail Treatment

Henna is a natural nail strengthener and conditioner. With just a few applications it will make your nails thicker, healthier, and stronger. Make sure you use colorless (neutral) henna or your nails will be dyed a soft red shade. Using henna to treat and color the nails was a popular practice in ancient Egypt. Centuries later, archaeologists have discovered mummies with beautiful red-tinted nails.

½ teaspoon neutral henna powder
½ cup boiling water

Mix together the henna powder and boiling water and stir well to dissolve the henna powder. *Do not use metal utensils or containers when mixing the henna.* Pour into a clean container with a tight-fitting lid.

Using a clean cotton swab, apply the henna solution to clean, dry nails and allow to dry. Repeat 2 or 3 times. This can be done every couple of days to keep your nails conditioned and strong.

Note: You may need to shake the henna solution before using to distribute the henna evenly.

Yield: 4 ounces

Castor Oil Nail Rub

2 teaspoons salt
2 teaspoons castor oil
1 teaspoon wheat germ oil

My mother's grandmother used to use castor oil as a health tonic. She would make her children take a tablespoonful whenever they looked a bit pale. It was also a very popular cosmetic oil (and still is), and was added to many creams, lotions, hair products, and lipsticks. In this recipe, castor oil is used to strengthen and shine the nails.

Combine all ingredients and mix thoroughly. Pour into a clean bottle with a lid. Shake before using.

Rub a small amount of the oil mixture into your nails, leave on for 3 to 5 minutes, and tissue off. Follow up with more castor oil rubbed into your nails if you wish.

Yield: ¾ ounce

Nail Whitener

2 tablespoons orange flower water
1 teaspoon fresh lemon juice

Sometimes your nails can be discolored from nail polish, cigarette smoke, paint, or other substances. This is a simple treatment for safely bleaching your nails back to their natural color.

Mix together the orange flower water and lemon juice. Pour into a clean container with a tight-fitting lid.

Using a clean cotton swab, apply the nail whitener to clean, dry nails and allow to dry. Repeat 2 or 3 times. This can be done every couple of days until your nails are back to their natural color. (Make sure you moisturize your hands and cuticles thoroughly, as the lemon juice can be drying.)

Yield: 1 ounce

Paraffin Hand Treatment

*H*ot wax treatments are used to plump up dry skin. First massage your hands with a good, rich hand cream or oil, then dip them in warm melted paraffin wax to help the cream penetrate into your hands. This treatment takes a little practice, and you may need help dipping your hands in the melted wax. If you like the idea of this treatment, but don't want to mess with melted wax, you may use heated rubber gloves (warmed by running hot water over them, taking care to keep the insides dry).

1 stick kitchen paraffin, about
   4 ounces
Your favorite rich hand cream or oil

Melt the paraffin wax in a double boiler or a heat-proof container in a pan of water on the stove top. When the wax is melted, remove from the heat and allow to cool. (I pour the wax into a pie tin, as this makes it easier to dip both my hands in it.)

Massage your hands with the hand cream. Test the wax by placing a small amount on your wrist—it should be warm, not hot. Dip your hands in the melted wax (some people prefer to brush the wax onto their hands; you may need help doing this). Allow the wax to cool and harden (20 to 30 minutes).

Peel the wax off your hands and discard. Massage any leftover cream into your hands and cuticles.

Note: You may use beeswax instead of paraffin if you prefer.

Yield: 4 ounces, 1 treatment

Fragrance

*F*ragrance is to your sense of smell as color is to your eyes—entertaining, exciting, and stimulating.

Perfumes and scents have been used throughout history, playing a significant role in people's lives as far back as the reign of King Menes, sometime around 3100 B.C. Fragrance has even been known to *make* history—and change it. The queen of Sheba used perfumes to seduce King Solomon. Cleopatra used scents to attract and influence the Greeks and Romans. Napoléon was known to have used more than sixty bottles of perfume each month.

The terms used in making fragrances resemble those used in making music. Septimus Piesse, a French chemist and perfumer, came up with the idea of combining perfumes into harmonies according to the musical scale. Each note had a scent. For example, A was lavender, B, peppermint, C, citronella, and so on. Today these terms are still used by perfume manufacturers. A fragrance is composed of three notes. The high note is the first scent your nose detects—citrus scents are almost always high notes. Middle notes determine the personality of the perfume—these tend to be floral scents. The low note is the scent that lingers on the skin or in the air after you depart—sandalwood, vanilla, and musk are all low notes. Great fragrance is like a beautiful chorus of delicate notes.

All fragrance falls into one of six basic scent groups. When choosing a scent, you may want to stay within a group or mix different groups to create your own unique scent. Remember that your own body chemistry plays an important role in how a particular fragrance will feel and smell on you.

Basic Scent Groups

Floral:	Rose, frangipani, jasmine, violet, lilac
Spice:	Cinnamon, ginger, cloves, allspice
Wood:	Pine, cedar, sandalwood
Fruit:	Lemon, orange, peach, coconut
Herbal:	Lavender, chamomile, sage, bay
Exotic:	Musk (herbal musk), orchid, ylang-ylang, vanilla

When making and testing new scents, never try more than three at a time. Your nose will lose its ability to tell the difference if exposed to too many scents at once.

Perfume and cologne are similar in composition; the main difference is in the percentage of alcohol and the amount of aromatic oils used. Cologne usually contains 1 to 2 percent aromatic oil, while perfume can contain up to 30 percent. Aromatic oils are also called essential oils, volatile oils, or essences, and are made from various parts of plants, flower petals, bark, leaves, and roots. These oils are removed from the plant at the prime of life; perhaps this is why man-made oils have failed in reproducing the qualities of these natural oils.

The recipes in this chapter are closer to colognes than perfumes. Perfumes are expensive to create because of their high percentage of aromatic oils. Homemade versions also do not have as long a shelf life as commercial ones. This is due to the use in commercial products of fixatives such as ambergris (from whales), civet (from the civet cats found in Ethiopia), and musk (from musk deer)—all of which are quite difficult to find. I prefer using glycerine, orrisroot powder, or castor oil as fixatives in my recipes.

Have fun experimenting with new and different scents. I like to have three scents around the house—a floral one for everyday wear, a heavy, spicy one for evening, and a light, fresh citrus one for outdoor activities and sports. Make small amounts of your perfumes and share them. Heat and light can affect your fragrances, so store them in clean, airtight containers and keep them in a cool, dark place. Colored jars and bottles work well to filter out light, which may alter the scent of your products. Do not use plastic containers, as this can sometimes alter the balance of the ingredients. Keep your containers as full as possible to avoid too much air contact; if need be, transfer to smaller containers. Your products should last about six months—longer, if you follow the steps outlined above.

Effleurage

1 small glass jar (6 to 8 ounces)
1 to 2 cups (enough to fill your glass
    jar several times) fresh flower
    petals (I like to use lavender, rose,
    lilac, and gardenia.)
1 cup light vegetable oil, such as
    sunflower or almond

Effleurage *is an age-old process used for making perfumed oils. Aromatic oils from flower petals are extracted, using the heat of the sun. The perfumed oil may be used alone or may be added as a scent to any of your favorite beauty recipes. (Layering scents is an effective way to use fragrance.) Use this perfumed oil in lotions, bath oils, and colognes as well.*

Fill a glass jar with the flower petals. Cover the petals with oil (it is all right if you do not use all the oil). Place the jar in a sunny spot. Let sit for 24 hours.

Strain off the oil and discard the flower petals. Add fresh flower petals and let sit for another 24 hours. Continue straining off oil and adding fresh flower petals for 3 or 4 days or until the oil has a scent you are pleased with. You may stabilize your fragrance (keep it from changing) after the scent has developed to your liking (4 or 5 days) by using one or two drops of glycerine, castor oil, or a pinch of orrisroot powder.

Store in a cool place in a clean, airtight container.

To use: Apply a small amount to your skin with a clean finger or cotton ball.

Note: To create an alcohol-based product from your scented oil: Take your *effleurage* and mix with an equal amount of alcohol (vodka). Let stand for a day, then shake. Do this every day for a week. The alcohol will absorb the scent from the oil (the *effleurage* oil will still have a scent).

Yield: approximately 6 to 8 ounces

Eau de Cologne

Eau de cologne *is French for "water of cologne." Originally it was made by steeping flowers in a jar with alcohol and a small amount of oil. The scented oil was poured off and the alcohol was mixed with water. Cologne water is perfect for daytime use, as it is lighter than perfume.*

¼ cup vodka
¼ cup water
2–3 drops of your favorite essential oil or a mixture of lavender, musk (herbal musk from musk seed, ambrette seed, musk mallow, or musk clover), sandalwood, bergamot, rose, frangipani, ylang-ylang, or jasmine

Mix all ingredients together. Pour into a clean spray bottle or splash bottle.

To use: Spray or splash the scented cologne onto the skin or hair.

Yield: 4 ounces

Hungary Water

A *very long time ago in Hungary there lived a queen named Maria who was known for her beauty and love of fragrance. Legend has it that she developed a fragrant orange water to entice and tantalize her many suitors. One young Polish king became so enamored with her that he proposed marriage—she was seventy-two at the time and he was only eighteen! There are many recipes for Hungary water. They all contain bergamot (orange), lavender, and citrus oils, but in a variety of proportions.*

⅛ teaspoon oil of orange (or lemon)
½ teaspoon bergamot oil
¼ teaspoon lavender oil
½ cup vodka
⅛ teaspoon glycerine or castor oil or orrisroot powder

Mix together all ingredients in a glass or ceramic container and cover with a lid or plastic wrap. Place in a cool, dark place and let sit for 1 week before using.

The best way to apply scents is by spraying them onto the skin, but you can also use your fingers to dab them on—especially at the pulse points (behind the ears, wrists, knees, inside the elbows).

Yield: 4 ounces

Victorian Handkerchief Cologne

1 tablespoon dried rosemary
1 tablespoon dried lavender flowers
5 whole allspice seeds
¼ cup vodka
⅛ teaspoon glycerine or castor oil or
   orrisroot powder

*U*nder Queen Victoria's reign in the mid-nineteenth to early twentieth century, Britain became a world power. During those years, ladies scented their handkerchiefs with perfumes and colognes and kept them tucked discreetly away—today, you can use this old-fashioned fragrance anywhere you wish!

Mix together all ingredients in a glass or ceramic container and cover with a lid or plastic wrap. Place in a cool, dark place and let sit for 1 week before using.

The best way to apply scents is by spraying them onto the skin, but you can also use your fingers to dab them on—especially at the pulse points (behind the ears, wrists, knees, inside the elbows).

Yield: 2 ounces

Irresistible Rose Cologne

½ cup dried rose petals (1½ cups
   fresh petals)
1 teaspoon dried orange peel
1 teaspoon dried lavender flowers
¼ cup vodka
⅛ teaspoon glycerine or castor oil or
   orrisroot powder

*R*oses have been revered for generations as a symbol of purity, faith, and beauty. Worldwide, their scent is one of the most recognizable and beloved. Use delicate rose petals from your garden or a friend's to make this enticing fragrance. Make sure you use fresh garden roses, as commercially grown roses do not have as strong a scent. In fact, many don't have any scent at all!

Mix together all ingredients in a glass or ceramic container and cover with a lid or plastic wrap. Place in a cool, dark place and let sit for 1 week before using.

The best way to apply scents is by spraying them onto the skin, but you can also use your fingers to dab them on—especially at the pulse points (behind the ears, wrists, knees, inside the elbows).

Yield: 2 ounces

Orchid Isle Cologne

On the big island of Hawaii I once stayed at a lovely hotel named the Orchid Isle. Hawaii is world renowned for the orchid plants that grow on the islands. I was captivated by the elegant beauty of these flowers. Vanilla beans come from orchid plants—a very exotic beginning for such a well-known and common scent! Vanilla has become a very popular ingredient in commercial perfumes today as a low or base note. If I've run out of this scent I sometimes just use straight vanilla extract from the grocery store—it's not as complex, but it's perfectly effective.

½ vanilla bean, split lengthwise
1 tablespoon dried rose petals
1 teaspoon orange peel
¼ cup vodka
⅛ teaspoon glycerine or castor oil or orrisroot powder

Mix together all ingredients in a glass or ceramic container and cover with a lid or plastic wrap. Place in a cool, dark place and let sit for 1 week before using.

The best way to apply scents is by spraying them onto the skin, but you can also use your fingers to dab them on—especially at the pulse points (behind the ears, wrists, knees, inside the elbows).

Yield: 2 ounces

Summer Garden Cologne

4 tablespoons fresh or 2 tablespoons
  dried rose petals
1 teaspoon fresh or ½ teaspoon dried
  citrus peel (orange, lemon, lime)
1 teaspoon fresh or ¼ teaspoon dried
  basil
1 teaspoon fresh or ¼ teaspoon dried
  rosemary
1 teaspoon fresh or ¼ teaspoon dried
  mint
¼ cup vodka
⅛ teaspoon glycerine or castor oil or
  orrisroot powder

In the summer I love to walk out into the garden and gather the ingredients for this fresh, light cologne. If you do not have fresh flowers and herbs growing in your yard—or if you don't have a yard—you may use the dried variety available at many natural food stores and farmers' markets.

Mix together all ingredients in a glass or ceramic container and cover with a lid or plastic wrap. Place in a cool, dark place and let sit for 1 week before using.

The best way to apply scents is by spraying them onto the skin, but you can also use your fingers to dab them on—especially at the pulse points (behind the ears, wrists, knees, inside the elbows).

Yield: 2 ounces

Mona Lisa Voile

¼ cup distilled water
⅛ teaspoon castor oil
6–8 drops essential oil of your choice

Mona Lisa's smile has what the French would call je ne sais quoi—*a quality that cannot be described but is beautiful. The word "voile" is French for "veil," a very light, delicate scent. Just a whisper of this fragrance on your skin eludes description. This recipe does not contain any alcohol, making it perfect for very dry skin.*

Mix together all ingredients and shake well. Pour into a clean spray container with a tight-fitting lid.

Always shake before using, then apply by spraying or splashing the scent on your skin.

Note: The 6 to 8 drops of essential oil is just a guideline; you may wish to add a little more or a little less to suit your own taste.

Yield: 2 ounces

Lavender Dry Perfume

*D*ry perfumes are similar to sachets. Nefertiti, queen of Egypt during the eighteenth dynasty, always carried her personal scent with her in a small pouch attached to her waist. Dry perfumes are more intense in scent than powders, and are used in place of perfume to scent the skin and hair.

1 teaspoon orrisroot powder
1 tablespoon dried lavender flowers
1 tablespoon cornstarch
2 drops lavender oil

Mix together all ingredients. Place the mixture in a food processor, blender, or coffee grinder and process until a smooth powder is achieved. (You may also use a mortar and pestle if you wish to grind the powder by hand.)

Place in a clean container with a tight-fitting lid. To apply, rub a small amount of this scented powder on your skin where you would apply perfume or cologne.

Yield: 1 ounce

Citrus Dry Perfume

1 teaspoon orrisroot powder
1 tablespoon cornstarch
1 tablespoon dried orange peel
2 drops lemon oil
2 drops bergamot oil

This recipe is similar to Lavender Dry Perfume (page 221) but has the fresh, fruity scent of citrus. Bergamot oil comes from oranges with the same name.

Mix together all ingredients. Place the mixture in a food processor, blender, or coffee grinder and process until a smooth powder is achieved. (You may also use a mortar and pestle if you wish to grind the powder by hand.)

Place in a clean container with a tight-fitting lid. To apply, rub a small amount of this scented powder on your skin where you would apply perfume or cologne.

Yield: 1 ounce

After-Bath Splash

¼ cup distilled water
¼ cup of your favorite cologne (see pages 217–220)

After-bath splashes are meant to be used liberally after bathing or any time you need a refreshing treat. They are lighter than colognes and not as potent. Their scents do not linger for as long, but they are a great way to start or end your day.

Mix together the water and cologne. Pour into a clean bottle with a tight-fitting stopper or spray nozzle.

Apply generously to your skin, especially after a bath or shower.

Yield: 4 ounces

Attar of Roses

Attar of roses is another name for the volatile oil contained inside the fresh petals, and it is used in making rose water and scented perfumes. Use only fresh petals that have been picked in the morning after the dew has evaporated but before the strong afternoon sun has warmed them.

2–3 cups fresh rose petals and leaves
Coarse salt such as kosher or rock salt

Gently wash the rose petals and leaves, and pat them dry between a layer of cotton towels or paper towels. Place a layer of the petals inside a clean ceramic crock or dark-colored glass jar. Over each layer sprinkle a thin covering of salt; repeat until the crock or jar is full. Cover your container tightly and place in a cool, dark spot for 3 to 6 weeks. The salt extracts the moisture from the petals and leaves, which should collect in the bottom of your jar. Strain the liquid through a coffee filter or several layers of cheesecloth. This is your scented attar of roses. To make fresh rose water, add a drop or two of this oil to 1 cup of distilled water.

Yield: 1–2 ounces

Solid Perfume

1 tablespoon grated beeswax
1 tablespoon almond oil
8 drops cologne or essential oil blend
   (see suggestions below)

FRUITY

3 drops peach oil, 3 drops sweet
   orange oil, 2 drops chamomile oil

SPICY

3 drops clove oil, 3 drops sandalwood
   oil, 2 drops cinnamon oil

EXOTIC

5 drops vanilla oil, 3 drops
   ylang-ylang oil

Solid perfume and scents have always been popular because they are long-lasting, easy to carry, and discreet—you can just rub them on and don't have to spray the air all around you. Throughout history great beauties such as Nefertiti, Cleopatra, Madame de Pompadour, and Irene Langhorne (the original Gibson Girl) carried their own personal scents, and now you can too. They are easy to make, and the procedures are basically the same as making a flavored lip balm. Pour your blends into vintage compacts or pillboxes for a unique package to slip into a pocket or purse. Any fragrance can be given a solid form—just remember that oil-based scents will last longer.

In a heat-resistant container or small saucepan, gently heat the beeswax and oil until the beeswax is melted. Stir in the scented oil or cologne and pour into a clean container with a lid. Allow the mixture to cool completely.

To use: Rub your finger across the solid perfume and apply the scent to your pulse points or wherever you wish.

Yield: 1 ounce

Lavender Linen Spray

½ cup distilled water
1 teaspoon vodka or witch hazel
5–6 drops essential oil of lavender

The scent of lavender is a classic for keeping linens fresh, warding off pests, and enhancing sleep and relaxation. Use this scented water in your iron when pressing fine linens to protect and freshen them. Spray generously onto your bed pillow each evening for a cradle-deep sleep.

Mix together all ingredients and pour into a clean spray bottle or glass container with a tight-fitting lid.

To use: Spray on your sheets and table linens before using or while pressing with a hot iron.

Yield: 4 ounces

Powders

*P*owder is used to absorb moisture and keep the skin feeling dry and comfortable. It also keeps you smelling fresh, as body odor is usually caused by bacteria that can grow in the moisture on the skin's surface. I like to use powder in hot weather to keep cool and comfortable, and I never put on a pair of shoes without a sprinkling of foot powder. After a bath, using powder from a big fluffy puff is a real treat for many women I know. You can also make your own shaker by punching holes in the lid of a jar, pouring your powder into the jar, and screwing on the lid.

Many commercial powders use talc, which is powdered soapstone or steatite. I have chosen to replace talc with cornstarch and rice flour in my recipes, since there has been some evidence recently that talc, like asbestos, may cause lung problems, especially in infants. There are also studies that have linked talc and ovarian cancer.

Powders are very simple to create and have a very long shelf life. I like to mix and keep my powders in airtight resealable plastic bags and jars. Store your powders in a dry place. The powders in this chapter are suitable for infants, children, and adults.

Chlorophyll

Lawn clippings, cut fine (I use
  scissors to cut the grass into
  small bits.)
1 cup vodka or witch hazel

Chlorophyll is known for its odor-absorbing properties and is used in many of my powder recipes. It will also give your mixtures a lovely green color. Chlorophyll can be found at most drugstores in liquid form, but it's just as easy to make your own, using lawn or grass clippings. (The majority of the chlorophyll sold commercially is derived from alfalfa grass.) Make sure the grass you use has not been treated with any chemicals, or these will end up in your chlorophyll solution.

Fill a clean, widemouthed jar with the lawn clippings. Pour the vodka over the clippings. Place the lid on the jar tightly. Set the jar in a cool, dark place for 1 week.

Strain off the liquid and discard the clippings. You now have liquid chlorophyll to use.

Yield: 8 ounces

Simple Bath Powder

½ cup cornstarch
½ cup rice flour

This is a simple recipe for a basic body powder. You could use ordinary cornstarch straight from the box for an even simpler powder. Mixing the cornstarch with a little rice flour gives it a more even texture, making it easier to smooth over the body.

Place the cornstarch and rice flour in a resealable jar, plastic bag, or container. Seal the container and shake gently until the powder is well mixed.

Apply the powder with a shaker-type container, or use a pretty jar with a powder puff.

Yield: 8 ounces

Scented Bath Powder

Scented powders make wonderful gifts and can be combined with lotions and colognes having similar scents. Once you have mastered this recipe, you can make powders to match all your favorite scents. Powders are perfect for this, as they absorb and hold fragrance very well.

1 cup cornstarch
5–6 drops of your favorite perfume or essential oil

There are two methods to choose from in mixing this powder, using a blender or a sealable container.

BLENDER METHOD:

Place the cornstarch in the blender and blend on low speed. With the blender still running, slowly add the perfume or oil. When well mixed, pour into a clean container.

You may apply with a shaker-type container, or use a pretty jar with a powder puff.

CONTAINER METHOD:

Place the cornstarch in a sealable jar, plastic bag, or container. Add the perfume or oil. Seal the container and shake gently until the powder is well mixed.

To use: Sprinkle the powder on your skin.

Yield: 8 ounces

Scented Rice Flour Powder

½ cup rice flour (white is preferred)
¼ cup cornstarch
1 tablespoon orrisroot powder (optional)
3–4 drops of your favorite essential oil or 1 teaspoon of your favorite cologne

*T*his is another version of Simple Bath Powder (page 228), with a few more ingredients. Rice flour is added to give the powder a smoother texture and make it easier to sprinkle on the skin. Orrisroot powder is used as a fixative to hold the scent a bit longer.

There are two methods to choose from in mixing this powder, using a blender or a sealable container.

BLENDER METHOD:

Place the rice flour, cornstarch, and orrisroot powder in the blender and start, blending the mixture on low. With the blender still running, slowly add the scented oil or cologne. When well mixed, pour into a clean container.

You may apply with a shaker-type container, or use a pretty jar with a powder puff.

CONTAINER METHOD:

Place the rice flour, cornstarch, and orrisroot powder in a resealable jar, plastic bag, or container. Add the scented oil or cologne. Seal the container and shake gently until the powder is well mixed.

You may apply with a shaker-type container, or use a pretty jar with a powder puff.

Note: You may need to add more scented oil or cologne if you wish a stronger scent.

Yield: 8 ounces

Almond Oil Powder

*A*dding a bit of almond oil, or any light oil, gives your powder a luxurious feel and softness. If you have dry skin, I would recommend this recipe. You may also substitute your favorite fragrance for the vanilla and almond extracts.

½ teaspoon vanilla extract
½ teaspoon almond extract
1 teaspoon almond oil (or any light oil)
1 cup cornstarch

There are two methods to choose from in mixing this powder, using a blender or a sealable container.

BLENDER METHOD:

Mix together the extracts and almond oil. Place the cornstarch in the blender and start blending it on low. With the blender still running, slowly add the oil mixture. When well mixed, pour into a clean container.

You may apply with a shaker-type container, or use a pretty jar with a powder puff.

CONTAINER METHOD:

Mix together the extracts and almond oil. Place the cornstarch in a resealable jar, plastic bag, or container. Add the oil mixture. Seal the container and shake gently until the powder is well mixed.

You may apply with a shaker-type container, or use a pretty jar with a powder puff.

Yield: 8 ounces

Peppermint Powder

½ teaspoon peppermint oil
1 teaspoon vodka or witch hazel
1 cup cornstarch

There is no denying the power of peppermint—it's an instant recharger! The peppermint oil in this recipe makes it refreshing and energizing, especially on a tired body. This powder is my favorite for hot, sticky days—it keeps me cool and smiling!

There are two methods to choose from in mixing this powder, using a blender or a sealable container.

BLENDER METHOD:

Mix together the peppermint oil and vodka. Place the cornstarch in the blender and start blending on low. With the blender still running, slowly add the peppermint mixture. When well mixed, pour into a clean container.

You may apply with a shaker-type container, or use a pretty jar with a powder puff.

CONTAINER METHOD:

Mix together the peppermint oil and vodka. Place the cornstarch in a resealable jar, plastic bag, or container. Add the peppermint mixture. Seal the container and shake gently until the powder is well mixed.

You may apply with a shaker-type container, or use a pretty jar with a powder puff.

Yield: 8 ounces

Orange-Flower Powder

Orange oil, or neroli, comes from the bitter orange tree, and helps to relieve anxiety and calm the nerves. To get a better night's sleep, use this powder in the evening before going to bed—the scent is very relaxing. For extra-pleasant dreams, sprinkle a bit on your sheets before getting into bed.

1 cup cornstarch
1 teaspoon orange flower water
2–3 drops orange oil (neroli)

There are two methods to choose from in mixing this powder, using a blender or a sealable container.

BLENDER METHOD:

Place the cornstarch in the blender and start blending on low. With the blender still running, slowly add the orange flower water and orange oil, one at a time. When well mixed, pour into a clean container.

You may apply with a shaker-type container, or use a pretty jar with a powder puff.

CONTAINER METHOD:

Place the cornstarch in a resealable jar, plastic bag, or container. Add the orange flower water and orange oil. Seal the container and shake gently until the powder is well mixed and the oil and water are dispersed.

You may apply to the skin with a shaker-type container, or use a pretty jar with a powder puff.

Yield: 8 ounces

Rose Geranium Powder

This is a wonderful, old-fashioned scented powder. Rose geraniums have the delicate scent of roses; the leaves are used in baking to make lovely perfumed tea cakes. They are also perfect for scenting powders and soaps. Geraniums are one of the most common and easy-to-grow indoor/outdoor plants. You may wish to purchase a small plant or take a cutting from a friend's garden.

1 cup cornstarch
1 teaspoon baking soda
5–6 fresh rose geranium leaves or
   2–3 drops rose geranium oil

Place the cornstarch and baking soda in a resealable jar, plastic bag, or container. Add the rose geranium leaves or oil. Seal the container, shake well, and let sit for 3 or 4 days, shaking it once a day.

Remove the leaves and discard. You now have a delicately scented powder to use and enjoy.

To use: Sprinkle the powder on your skin.

Yield: 8 ounces

Violet Powder

Orrisroot is known for its delicate violet scent. The ancient Egyptians and Greeks discovered that this bland-smelling root of the iris flower would take on a remarkable fragrance when dried and aged. The aromatic powers of orrisroot increase with age; fresh orrisroot actually has very little fragrance.

1 cup cornstarch
1 tablespoon dried orrisroot powder
2–3 drops oil of orris (optional)

Place the cornstarch and orrisroot powder in a sealable jar, plastic bag, or container. Add the orris oil if you wish a stronger scent. Seal the container and shake gently until the powder is well mixed.

To use: Sprinkle the powder on your skin.

Yield: 8 ounces

Deodorant Powder

This is a simple but effective deodorant powder. Body odor is caused by perspiration and bacteria; keeping the body dry and preventing odor-causing bacteria will help to eliminate body odor. This powder is perfect to use after a bath, a shower, or exercise. For best results, apply to clean, dry skin.

1 cup cornstarch
1 tablespoon baking soda
1 teaspoon liquid chlorophyll

There are two methods to choose from in mixing this powder, using a blender or a sealable container.

BLENDER METHOD:

Place the cornstarch and baking soda in the blender and blend the mixture on low. With the blender still running, slowly add the chlorophyll. When well mixed, pour into a clean container.

You may apply with a shaker-type container, or use a pretty jar with a powder puff.

CONTAINER METHOD:

Place the cornstarch and baking soda in a resealable jar, plastic bag, or container. Add the chlorophyll. Seal the container and shake gently until the powder is well mixed and the chlorophyll is dispersed.

You may apply with a shaker-type container, or use a pretty jar with a powder puff.

Yield: 8 ounces

Carmen Miranda Fruit Powder

½ cup rice flour
½ cup cornstarch
1 tablespoon orrisroot powder
   (optional)
4–5 drops essential oil, either alone or
   in combination: lemon, orange,
   peach, coconut, strawberry

Carmen Miranda, the popular 1940s movie star, often wore big baskets of fruit on her head. This is a powder recipe that Carmen would have loved. Strawberry and lemon have always been popular scents, and you can experiment with other fruit fragrances such as peach or coconut or a combination.

There are two methods to choose from in mixing this powder, using a blender or a sealable container.

BLENDER METHOD:

Place the rice flour, cornstarch, and orrisroot powder in the blender and blend the mixture on low. With the blender still running, slowly add the essential oil. When well mixed, pour into a clean container.

You may apply with a shaker-type container, or use a pretty jar with a powder puff.

CONTAINER METHOD:

Place the rice flour, cornstarch, and orrisroot powder in a sealable jar, plastic bag, or container. Add the essential oil. Seal the container and shake gently until the powder is well mixed.

You may apply with a shaker-type container, or use a pretty jar with a powder puff.

Note: You may need to add more oil if you wish a stronger scent.

Yield: 8 ounces

Cloud Nine Powder

A sprinkling of this powder on your feet will make you feel as though you're walking on cloud nine. When you don't want to wear socks in the summer, this powder helps to absorb moisture and perspiration. Rub a bit into tired feet at the end of the day to refresh and revive them.

2 tablespoons rice flour
2 tablespoons cornstarch
1 tablespoon baking soda
½ teaspoon orrisroot powder
   (optional)
3 drops essential oil of geranium

There are two methods to choose from in mixing this powder, using a blender or a sealable container.

BLENDER METHOD:

Place the rice flour, cornstarch, baking soda, and orrisroot powder in the blender and blend the mixture on low. With the blender still running, slowly add the essential oil. When well mixed, pour into a clean container.

You may apply with a shaker-type container.

CONTAINER METHOD:

Place the rice flour, cornstarch, baking soda, and orrisroot powder in a sealable jar, plastic bag, or container. Add the essential oil. Seal the container and shake gently until the powder is well mixed.

Apply a small amount to your feet and massage in. You may also want to sprinkle a bit inside your shoes.

Note: You may need to add more oil if you wish a stronger scent.

Yield: 3 ounces

Cooling Cinnamon Powder

½ cup cornstarch
1 tablespoon ground cinnamon

Heat rash or prickly heat can occur any time conditions prevent perspiration from evaporating. It is especially common in the summer months; when the weather is hot and humid people tend to perspire more. The best way to prevent heat rash is to stay cool. Choose light clothing made from natural fibers such as cotton, linen, or silk. You may also want to use cornstarch as a body powder. Try this cinnamon-scented body powder to stay cool and dry.

Mix together the cornstarch and cinnamon until thoroughly blended. Then pour the mixture into a clean, dry jar with a few holes punched in the lid.

To use: Sprinkle the powder on your skin before dressing, or over your bedsheets for a good night's sleep.

Yield: 4 ounces

Mouthwashes and Tooth Powders

Smile and the whole world smiles with you! The most important thing you can do for your mouth is to keep your teeth and gums really clean. I am a firm believer in regularly brushing the teeth and gums. It is one of the easiest and best preventive steps you can take for a healthy mouth. Mouthwashes kill bacteria in the mouth, strengthen the gums, and help keep your breath fresh.

When I was in college I was asked to give a speech on a socially significant issue. I chose halitosis. My speech professor was not amused, but I did get an A. The following tips for avoiding bad breath are from that college speech:

1. Eat regular meals. Ever wonder why people who are constantly dieting often have bad breath? This is caused by bacteria that build up in the stomach between meals.

2. Brush your tongue and gums, as well as your teeth.

3. Floss your teeth at least once a day—before going to bed is best.

4. Brush your teeth after every meal.

5. Drink plenty of water throughout the day to keep your mouth well hydrated.

Mouthwashes and tooth powders will keep for quite a long time. Mouthwashes contain alcohol or acids, which help to kill germs and bacteria. Tooth powders will last until you use them up as long as they are kept dry. They should be kept in airtight containers so they don't attract odors.

Herb Garden Mouthwash

2 tablespoons fresh parsley
2 tablespoons fresh mint
1 cup distilled water
1 tablespoon vodka (optional)

Two of nature's most effective mouth-freshening herbs are parsley and mint, both of which kill bacteria in the mouth and reduce bad breath. I like to use this mouthwash full strength twice a day, in the morning and at night. It tastes sort of like an herb garden cocktail—green and grassy. I would not recommend swallowing it (but it would not harm you if you did).

Combine all ingredients in a blender and process on high until well blended (about 2 minutes). Pour the liquid through a strainer into a clean container.

To use: Pour about 4 teaspoons into a glass and rinse your mouth for 30 seconds. Do not swallow—it is safe to drink, but it does contain alcohol (vodka).

Yield: 8 ounces

Rose Water Mouthwash

1 tablespoon vodka (optional)
2 tablespoons rose water
1 cup distilled water

This is a mild, almost tasteless rinse with the delicate fragrance of roses. It also works as a skin freshener and an after-bath splash. Because it's so versatile, it's a good product to pack when traveling. If you prefer a mouthwash without alcohol, simply omit the vodka in this recipe. Rose water itself has mild antiseptic properties that act in killing germs.

Combine all ingredients and pour into a clean bottle. Shake well to mix.

To use: Pour about 4 teaspoons into a glass and rinse your mouth for 30 seconds.

Yield: 9½ ounces

Clove Mouthwash

Evergreen clove trees thrive in warm climates such as Madagascar, India, and the Philippines. The unopened flower buds are well known as a temporary cure for toothaches because of their mildly anesthetic properties. This mouthwash is a good rinse to use if you have sensitive teeth or gums. Cloves have a sharp, distinctive flavor. In this recipe, you may use ground cloves or clove oil (sold in many pharmacies). The oil can be made at home by soaking a few whole cloves in a tablespoon of olive oil overnight.

¼ cup vodka
½ cup distilled water
¼ teaspoon honey
¼ teaspoon cinnamon
½ teaspoon ground cloves or clove oil

Combine all the ingredients and stir well until all the honey is dissolved. Pour into a clean bottle. You may also want to filter the mouthwash if you have used ground cloves, to remove the clove pieces.

To use: Pour about 4 teaspoons into a glass and rinse your mouth for 30 seconds.

Yield: 5 ounces

Strawberry Leaf Mouth Rinse

Eating fresh strawberries will whiten and clean your teeth by removing plaque. This is due to the berries' high content of salicylic acid. The leaves make an effective mouthwash because they also have antiseptic properties. This recipe is perfect for those who do not wish to use alcohol but want a clean mouth.

¼ cup dried or 1 cup fresh strawberry
    leaves
1 cup boiling water
2 teaspoons fresh lemon juice

Place the strawberry leaves in a ceramic bowl and pour the boiling water over them. Let sit until completely cool. Strain off the liquid and discard the leaves. Add the lemon juice and stir well. Store this mouthwash in the refrigerator.

To use: Pour about 4 teaspoons into a glass and rinse your mouth for 30 seconds.

Yield: 8 ounces

NATURAL MOUTH FRESHENERS

The following is a list of natural mouth fresheners. Keep a small container of fennel seeds or dried ginger in your purse or briefcase for a quick breath freshener. When eating out, always eat the parsley or mint garnish. Some nutritionists say that eating these mouth fresheners is also good for the stomach, where mouth odors are believed to originate.

Parsley

Mint

Gingerroot

Fennel seeds

Basil

Anise seeds

Thyme

Juniper berries

Salt Water Rinse

This old-fashioned mouth rinse is simple, inexpensive, and sure to cure just about everything. When I was a child, my mother always made us gargle with warm salt water when we had sore throats. My dentist always recommends salt water for healing sore gums and to rid the mouth of bacteria.

1 cup warm water
1 teaspoon salt

Mix together the water and the salt. Stir until the salt is completely dissolved. Rinse the mouth and gargle with the mixture.

Note: This rinse works best when warm.

Yield: 8 ounces

TOOTH POWDERS

Tooth powders are popular dentifrices today because they are not as abrasive as many commercial toothpastes and many do not contain additives such as sudsing agents (hard soaps and detergents), binders, and artificial flavorings. They are also very inexpensive to make. Try to brush your teeth for at least two full minutes—place an egg timer next to your bathroom sink to keep track of the time.

Classic: Baking soda is the classic basic tooth powder because it is a mild abrasive and is very effective in cleaning the teeth and gums. Dip a damp toothbrush in a dish of baking soda and massage your teeth and gums.

Baking soda and salt: Mix together equal amounts of baking soda and table salt to create a gentle, cleansing tooth powder. Salt alone can be too abrasive, especially for sensitive teeth and gums.

Sage: Sage is a natural tooth whitener. Mixed with baking soda and salt, this powder will keep your whole mouth fresh and clean. Mix together a teaspoon each of dried sage, table salt, and baking soda.

Powdered orange peel: Dried orange peel that has been finely ground makes a good tooth powder with a mild citrus flavor. Use only the orange part, or zest, of the peel.

Soothing Tooth Powder

1 tablespoon arrowroot powder
1 teaspoon salt
½ teaspoon baking soda
Peppermint extract (optional)

This tooth powder is especially soothing to sensitive teeth and gums because it contains arrowroot, a fine, white powder that was used by Native Americans to heal arrow wounds. It can be found in many grocery stores and is similar to cornstarch in appearance, texture, and its use in cooking.

Mix together the arrowroot powder, salt, and baking soda. You may want to add a few drops of peppermint extract to make the powder taste a little less salty. Dip a damp toothbrush into this powder and brush your teeth.

Yield: 1½ ounces

Lavender Mouth Rinse

Lavender leaves freshen the breath and clean and disinfect the gums. This is a mild, almost tasteless mouth rinse that has an airy floral fragrance. You can also use this as a skin freshener or after-bath splash. This is especially helpful when you are traveling and you want to avoid carrying several different products. Both lavender and rose water are naturally antiseptic.

1 tablespoon lavender leaves
1 cup boiling water
2 tablespoons rose water

Place the lavender leaves in a glass or ceramic dish and pour the boiling water over them. Let this mixture steep for several hours, then strain and discard the leaves. Add the rose water to the scented liquid. Stir well and pour into a clean bottle.

To use: Pour a small amount into a clean glass and rinse your mouth after brushing your teeth and gums.

Yield: 8 ounces

Peppermint Toothpaste

The cool, clean taste of peppermint is a classic toothpaste flavor. This pale-colored gel is made using fresh mint leaves and will help clean both your teeth and gums. It is nonabrasive, making it a good choice for people with sensitive teeth and gums.

1 tablespoon fresh peppermint or ½
    tablespoon dried
¼ cup cold water
½ teaspoon sunflower oil
½ teaspoon cornstarch

Place the mint leaves and water in a small saucepan or microwave-safe container. Bring the mixture to a boil, remove from heat, and allow the mixture to cool for 15 to 20 minutes. Mix together the cornstarch and oil, and stir until smooth. Strain the mint-leaf solution and discard the leaves. Mix together the mint water and cornstarch mixture. Bring this mix to a boil and then cool, stirring occasionally. Spoon the cooled mixture into a clean container.

To use: Spread a small amount on a clean toothbrush and brush as usual.

Yield: 2 ounces

HEALTHY SMILE

Clean teeth and a great smile are beauty assets. Examine the "before" and "after" pictures in any magazine makeover and the "afters" always have a great smile and look much better. Here are some simple teeth-cleaning pointers to keep you smiling:

- **Use a supersoft brush:** A hard-bristle brush will push your gums back, which could cause infection. If your brush is too harsh, run it under hot water for a few minutes to soften the bristles.

- **Hold your toothbrush lightly:** If you grip your brush too tightly you may overscrub and damage your gums.

- **Don't brush up and down:** Brush in a circular motion first, to loosen bacteria and food particles. For your last few strokes, brush from the base of your gums in the direction your teeth grow.

- **Brush for two minutes:** Move the egg timer into the bathroom if you have to.

- **Brush or scrape your tongue:** A significant cause of bad breath is odor-causing bacteria on your tongue.

- **Floss!:** Always follow up your toothbrush session with dental floss for healthy teeth and gums.

Soap and
Soap Making

*S*oap is the oldest of all cleaning products. Before Procter and Gamble came along, people made their own soap and were quite serious about it—soap-making get-togethers were a part of pioneer life. Soap making is a simple process, using very basic ingredients, but it requires complete concentration, time, patience, and practice. It's very satisfying to use your own homemade soaps, and nothing smells or feels quite as clean. They also make unique gifts for friends and family.

There are many good books on soap and soap making, and some community centers offer soap-making classes. The best way to learn about making soap is to keep practicing. I don't want to tell you what my first soap looked like, but I can assure you it wasn't a lovely white bar.

The two basic ingredients for making soap are *fat* and *lye*. Fat can be derived from a number of sources—beef fat, or tallow, and vegetable oils are the most common. Lye, or caustic soda, can be found in the plumbing section in any hardware or grocery store. Only use products that are 100 percent lye for soap making. You can also purchase lye from chemical supply houses under the name of sodium hydroxide, but it is more expensive. *Always handle lye with extreme care—it can cause severe burns.*

The chemical process for making soap is called saponification, and the key to its success is temperature. The lye, mixed with cold water, must cool down to a certain temperature (when lye is mixed with water, the temperature rises to over 200° F.), and the fat/oils must be heated up to a certain temperature.

When the temperatures are right, the oil is saponified into soap by the lye. This process can take hours or even days; good soap is best if aged for at least a month.

The recipes I have included in this chapter are basic soaps to help you get started in the art of soap making. Read through the recipes carefully, and make sure you have all the ingredients before beginning. Be sure to follow the basic care and storage guidelines found on page 8.

SOAP-MAKING EQUIPMENT

You will need some special equipment dedicated entirely to soap making. Garage sales and flea markets are good sources for soap-making equipment.

Candy thermometers: One is enough, but two work best—one for the fat mixture and one for the lye solution.

Large enamel or steel pot: Do not use aluminum or iron as it reacts with the lye.

Large heat-resistant glass bottle or pitcher: For making the lye solution (around 40 ounces; many fruit juice bottles are this size). I have found that a large, heat-resistant jar, with two holes poked in the lid with an ice pick, makes an excellent container for the lye solution. The holes make pouring the solution in a steady stream easier.

Wooden spoons or paddles with long handles: For stirring.

Soap molds: Old muffin tins, loaf pans, large candy molds, even cardboard boxes work. The soap is more easily removed if the mold is oiled and lined with wax paper or with cotton cloth dipped in cold water and wrung dry. I like to use old muffin tins as they make round bars of soap.

Rubber gloves: To protect your hands.

BASIC SOAP-MAKING RULES

1. Always wear rubber gloves and protective clothing—long-sleeved shirts, long pants, and shoes.

2. Work in a well-ventilated area.

3. Keep some vinegar nearby to rub on skin if lye gets on it. Vinegar will neutralize the lye. *Remember: Lye is a poison and it burns!*

4. Always use *cold* water when mixing the lye solution.

5. Avoid all distractions—soap making requires attention to detail.

6. Use a thermometer to monitor oil and lye temperatures. (Below is a list of temperature guidelines; check individual recipes for suggested temperatures.)

7. Always pour the lye solution into the fat or oil mixture, not the other way around.

INGREDIENT TEMPERATURES FOR SOAP MAKING

Type of Fat	Fat Temperature	Lye Temperature
Tallow	120°–130° F.	90°–95° F.
Tallow and Lard	100°–110° F.	80°–85° F.
Lard/Vegetable Oils	80°–85° F.	70°–75° F.

Tallow Soap

FOR 9 POUNDS OF SOAP

6 pounds clean fat (about 13 cups)
¼ cup borax (optional)
1 13-ounce can lye granules
1½ pints water

FOR 1 BAR OF SOAP

1 cup clean fat
1 teaspoon borax (optional)
5 teaspoons lye granules
½ cup water

When I first began to experiment with making my own soaps, I wrote to the United States Department of Agriculture and asked for any recipes they might have. This is the recipe they sent me, and it makes a good basic bar of soap. Tallow, or fat, can be obtained from a variety of sources. I like to collect clean fat at home as I cook (before cooking, trim off clean beef or pork fat) and save it in the freezer until I am ready to make soap. You can also get it from your butcher or from tallow shops. The addition of borax is not necessary, although it can improve the appearance and lathering action of the soap.

Measure the clean fat. Heat slowly until completely melted, and then cool to approximately 110° F. Add borax if desired. Stir the fat occasionally during cooling.

Dissolve the lye in the water and cool to about 85° F. Pour the lye solution into the fat, pouring slowly in a thin, steady stream with slow, even stirring. You should not be applying any heat to the mixture at this time. Continue stirring until a thick, honeylike texture is obtained. This should take about 10 to 20 minutes.

(Note: If the soap mixture does not become thick within 30 minutes, and there is a greasy layer on top, it may be too warm. In this case, set the container in cool water and keep stirring from the sides and bottom. On the other hand, if the mixture is lumpy, it may be too cold. If this happens, set it in a pan of warm water and stir until the lumps disappear.)

Pour the thickened soap mixture into your molds. Cover and keep warm for at least 24 hours; this allows the saponification process to take place slowly and will prevent the mixture from separating. I wrap my soap molds in an old blanket.

Remove the soap and cut into bars. Allow the soap to age for at least 2 weeks in a dry place.

Note: If the soap is crumbly or has streaks of grease, it may be reclaimed as follows: Cut the soap into fine pieces, add water (7 pints for the large recipe and 1 cup for the small), and dissolve over low heat. Stir occasionally. When the lumps have disappeared, increase the heat and boil until the soap appears thick. Pour soap in molds and proceed as outlined above.

Basic Castile Soap

The Castile region of Spain is known for its production of fine olive oil. Soap given the Castile name must contain 40 percent olive oil. You will see this soap sold in many natural food and health food stores in both liquid and bar form. It is especially mild and gentle because it is made from vegetable products. I use this soap on my own skin as well as my daughters'—you can also use it to wash your hair.

2 cups olive oil
½ cup lye granules
2 cups cold water

Heat the olive oil slowly to approximately 80°–85° F. Dissolve the lye in the water and cool to about 70°–75° F.

Pour the lye solution into the oil, pouring slowly in a thin, steady stream with slow, even stirring. You should not be applying any heat to the mixture at this time. Continue stirring until a thick, honeylike texture is obtained. This should take about 10 to 20 minutes.

(Note: If the soap mixture does not become thick within 30 minutes, and there is a greasy layer on top, it may be too warm. In this case, set the container in cool water and keep stirring from the sides and bottom. On the other hand, if the mixture is lumpy, it may be too cold. If this happens, set it in a pan of warm water and stir until the lumps disappear.)

Pour the thickened soap mixture into your molds. Cover and keep warm for at least 24 hours; this allows the saponification process to take place slowly and will prevent the mixture from separating. I wrap my soap molds in an old blanket.

When the soap is set, remove from the molds and cut into bars. Allow the soap to age for at least 2 weeks in a dry place.

Note: If the soap is crumbly or has streaks of grease, it may be reclaimed as follows: Cut the soap into fine pieces, add 2 cups water, and dissolve over low heat. Stir occasionally. When the lumps have disappeared, increase the heat and boil until the soap appears thick. Pour soap in molds and proceed as outlined above.

Yield: approximately 12 2-ounce bars (depending on the mold you use)

Coconut Oil Soap

½ cup light vegetable oil
½ cup coconut oil
1 cup vegetable shortening
½ cup lye granules
2 cups cold water

Coconut oil is one of the most commonly used ingredients in commercial soap. It is added to many cleaning products because it increases their foaming, or sudsing, action. Like Basic Castile Soap (see page 255), this is also an all-vegetable soap and very mild—you can even use it to clean your lingerie.

Heat the oils and shortening slowly to approximately 80°–85° F.

Dissolve the lye in the water and cool to about 70°–75° F. Pour the lye solution into the oil mixture, pouring slowly in a thin, steady stream with slow, even stirring. You should not be applying any heat to the mixture at this time. Continue stirring until a thick, honeylike texture is obtained. This should take about 10 to 20 minutes.

(Note: If the soap mixture does not become thick within 30 minutes, and there is a greasy layer on top, it may be too warm. In this case, set the container in cool water and keep stirring from the sides and bottom. On the other hand, if the mixture is lumpy, it may be too cold. If this happens, set it in a pan of warm water and stir until the lumps disappear.)

Pour the thickened soap mixture into your molds. Cover and keep warm for at least 24 hours; this allows the saponification process to take place slowly and will prevent the mixture from separating. I wrap my soap molds in an old blanket.

When the soap is set, remove from the molds and cut into bars. Allow the soap to age for at least 2 weeks in a dry place.

Note: If the soap is crumbly or has streaks of grease, it may be reclaimed as follows: Cut the soap into fine pieces, add 2 cups water, and dissolve over low heat. Stir occasionally. When the lumps have disappeared, increase the heat and boil until the soap appears thick. Pour soap into molds and proceed as outlined above.

Yield: approximately 12 2-ounce bars (depending on the mold you use)

Cold-Cream Soap

1 cup light vegetable oil
1 cup vegetable shortening
½ cup lye granules
2 cups cold water
¼ cup cold cream (see Basic Cold
  Cream, page 63)

I *like to add a little cold cream when making soap for myself; it makes the end product less drying to my skin. Add the cream to the soap mixture after it has saponified and while it is cooling. You may use this same technique in other recipes if you wish.*

Heat the oil and shortening slowly to approximately 80°–85° F.

Dissolve the lye in the water and cool to about 70°–75° F. Pour the lye solution into the oil mixture, pouring slowly in a thin, steady stream with slow, even stirring. You should not be applying any heat to the mixture at this time. Continue stirring until a thick, honeylike texture is obtained. This should take about 10 to 20 minutes.

Add the cold cream and stir until well mixed.

(Note: If the soap mixture does not become thick within 30 minutes, and there is a greasy layer on top, it may be too warm. In this case, set the container in cool water and keep stirring from the sides and bottom. On the other hand, if the mixture is lumpy, it may be too cold. If this happens, set it in a pan of warm water and stir until the lumps disappear.)

Pour the thickened soap mixture into your molds. Cover and keep warm for at least 24 hours; this allows the saponification process to take place slowly and will prevent the mixture from separating. I wrap my soap molds in an old blanket.

When the soap is set, remove from the molds and cut into bars. Allow the soap to age for at least 2 weeks in a dry place.

Note: If the soap is crumbly or has streaks of grease, it may be reclaimed as follows: Cut the soap into fine pieces, add 2 cups water, and dissolve over low heat.

Stir occasionally. When the lumps have disappeared, increase the heat and boil until the soap appears thick. Pour soap into molds and proceed as outlined above.

Yield: 24 ounces, or 12 2-ounce bars (depending on the molds you use)

Oatmeal Soap

Oatmeal has long been added to soaps to give them extra texture, helpful in removing surface dirt and impurities. My grandmothers always used oatmeal to keep their skin clean and soft. The following recipe is for a tallow-based oatmeal soap. I have found cornmeal to work equally well in this recipe; just substitute it in place of the oatmeal.

1 cup clean fat
1 teaspoon borax powder (optional)
5 teaspoons lye granules
½ cup cold water
¼ cup oatmeal

Measure the clean fat. Heat slowly until completely melted, and cool to approximately 110° F. Add borax if desired, and stir the fat occasionally during cooling.

Dissolve the lye in the water, and cool to about 85° F. Pour the lye solution into the fat, pouring slowly in a thin, steady stream with slow, even stirring. You should not be applying any heat to the mixture at this time. Continue stirring until a thick, honeylike texture is obtained. This should take about 10 to 20 minutes. Add the oatmeal and stir until well mixed.

(Note: If the soap mixture does not become thick within 30 minutes, and there is a greasy layer on top, it may be too warm. In this case, set the container in cool water and keep stirring from the sides and bottom. On the other hand, if the mixture is lumpy, it may be too cold. If this happens, set it in a pan of warm water and stir until the lumps disappear.)

Pour the thickened soap mixture into your molds. Cover and keep warm for at least 24 hours. I wrap my soap molds in an old blanket.

Remove the soap by turning the mold over and gently tapping it on a counter or tabletop, and cut into bars. Allow the soap to age for at least 2 weeks in a dry place.

Note: If the soap is crumbly or has streaks of grease, it may be reclaimed as follows: Cut the soap into fine pieces, add 1 cup water, and dissolve over low heat. Stir occasionally. When the lumps have disappeared, increase the heat and boil until the soap appears thick. Pour soap into molds and proceed as outlined above.

Yield: 10 ounces, or 2 to 4 bars of soap (depending on mold size)

Glycerine Soap

2 cups light vegetable oil or fat or a
   combination of fat and oils
½ cup lye granules
2 cups cold water
½ cup glycerine

Glycerine is found naturally in many plants and is also a by-product of soap making. After the lye solution and the fat or oils are saponified, there is a clear, thick liquid that floats on top of the mixture—this is glycerine. It is a well-known humectant (a product that helps retain moisture). Glycerine soap is simply soap that has extra glycerine added to it shortly after the lye solution has been added. This recipe creates a mild soap that is very gentle on the skin.

Heat the oils and/or fat slowly to approximately 80°–85° F.

Dissolve the lye in the water and cool to about 70°–75° F. Pour the lye solution into the oil mixture, pouring slowly in a thin, steady stream with slow, even stirring. You should not be applying any heat to the mixture at this time. Slowly add the glycerine to the mixture and continue stirring until a thick, honeylike texture is obtained. This should take about 10 to 20 minutes.

(Note: If the soap mixture does not become thick within 30 minutes, and there is a greasy layer on top, it may be too warm. In this case, set the container in cool water and keep stirring from the sides and bottom. On the other hand, if the mixture is lumpy, it may be too cold. If this happens, set it in a pan of warm water and stir until the lumps disappear.)

Pour the thickened soap mixture into your molds. Cover and keep warm for at least 24 hours. I wrap my soap molds in an old blanket.

When the soap is set, remove from the molds and cut into bars. Allow the soap to age for at least 2 weeks in a dry place.

Note: If the soap is crumbly or has streaks of grease, it may be reclaimed as follows: Cut the soap into fine pieces, add 2 cups water, and dissolve over low heat. Stir occasionally. When the lumps have disappeared, increase the heat and boil until the soap appears thick. Pour soap into molds and proceed as outlined above.

Yield: 24 ounces, or 12 2-ounce bars (depending on the molds you use)

Super-Easy Oatmeal Soap

1 cup grated castile soap (1 3-ounce bar will yield this amount.)
¼ cup water
2 tablespoons oatmeal

If you want to create your own soaps, but don't want to bother with the complete soap-making process, this is the recipe for you! I take already-made castile soap (any mild soap will do) and add oatmeal to it—it makes an easy and very personal gift. Try substituting cornmeal or lavender flowers in place of the oatmeal as a variation.

Place the grated soap in a double boiler or ceramic bowl in a pan of water on the stove top. Pour the water over the soap and stir over medium heat to dissolve all of the soap in the water. When the soap and water are combined, add the oatmeal and stir well.

Pour the mixture into a greased mold. (I coat the mold with petroleum jelly, but you could also use vegetable shortening.) Let cool completely and unmold by turning the mold over and gently tapping it on a table or countertop. Let the soap dry for a few days.

Yield: 8 ounces, 1 large bar or 4 smaller ones

SOME VARIATIONS TO TRY IN
SOAP MAKING

Make it float: Almost any soap can be made to float. When the soap mixture is thick enough, use an electric mixer and "whip" the mixture to add air to it.

Perfume soap: If you want your soap to have a scent, mix in your favorite perfume oil or essential oil (after the mixture has cooled a bit and before you pour it into the molds). Never use perfume that contains alcohol—the scent will not last as long and it may cause separation in your soap mixture. Soaps absorb odors, and you can scent your soaps inexpensively by placing them in a box with petals and leaves from your favorite flowers. (Rose geranium leaves make a lovely scented soap.)

Colored soap: You can purchase dyes to use in soap making, or make your own using vegetables and spices. For example, a red color can be had by pounding the tops of beetroots to extract a few drops of the juice. Yellow can be obtained from saffron or turmeric, and green from liquid chlorophyll (see page 228). The color can be added to the lye-water solution before it is poured into the fat or oil mixture.

Liquid soap: Any soap can be made into a liquid simply by dissolving it in water. I like to use a ratio of one part water to one part soap. For a thicker liquid, add less water or more soap; for a thinner liquid, add more water. You may also want to add a tablespoon of glycerine for every cup of liquid soap—it acts as a humectant, keeping water in the soap mixture.

(continued)

> **Flowers and herbs:** Mixing in dried flowers and herbs, such as rose petals, lavender, chamomile, mint, or basil, can make your soap look and smell even prettier. Just add one or two tablespoons to the soap mixture before pouring it into the molds, and stir well.

Soap Treasures

Coconut oil or vegetable shortening
1–2 bars glycerine soap
Small "treasures"

Soap making has become so popular that you can now very easily create boutique-style soaps at home with amazing results. One popular style of soap found in many shops and spas is a clear glycerine cake with objects visible inside. I like to call them "treasure" soaps because as you use your bar of soap the small object inside slowly appears. You can choose a variety of small objects to place inside your soap. Just make sure it can get wet and is not sharp. I like to use small plastic rings, necklaces, figures, slices of loofah sponge, dried flowers, herbs, and spices. They also make great holiday gifts and guest soaps — imagine spider rings for Halloween, golf tees for a big tournament, "superstar" necklaces for all your girlfriends.

I use cheap glycerine soap from the drugstore. You can also purchase loaves of glycerine soap at many craft stores. Some of the larger craft-store chains have aisles of soap-making equipment, soap, molds, and dyes for inspiration.

For soap molds I use plastic PVC pipe caps from the hardware store. You can also use measuring cups, candy molds, ice cube trays, cookie cutters (put foil over one side) to create fun and interesting shapes.

Grease your soap molds with coconut oil or vegetable shortening. With a knife, chop up your soap bars and place them in a heat-resistant container. Heat gently in the microwave or on the stove top until completely melted. Fill each of your soap molds halfway with the liquid soap. Let the soap harden (you can place it in the refrigerator to speed up this process). Place your small object on top of the hardened soap and fill the mold with more melted soap. Let the soap harden completely and then unmold. Use as you would any bar of soap.

Yield: 8 ounces, enough for 2 bars of soap, depending on size

Easy Soap Balls

I remember my grandmother always had soap balls in her guest bath, and I loved using them because of their smooth round shape. This old-fashioned recipe makes a soapy dough that can be shaped into balls or any shape that you like. Even children will have fun creating these easy-to-make special guest soaps.

2 cups gentle soap flakes (like grated
    Ivory soap)
¼ to ½ cup water
A few drops of food coloring
    (optional)
A few drops scented oil (optional)

Mix the soap flakes and water together until you have a smooth paste. You can do this by hand or use an electric mixer for lighter, fluffier soap dough. You may need to increase the water or soap until you have a smooth mixture. Add a few drops of food coloring if you wish to color your soap mixture. Then blend in a few drops of scented oil and mix well. Lightly coat your hands with some vegetable oil and mold the soap mixture into small balls. Place the soap on a sheet of waxed paper and let it harden for several hours.

    To use: Enjoy as you would any bar of soap in the tub, shower, or next to the sink.

Yield: 12 ounces, 4 average-size balls

Loofah Soap

2 bars of pure natural soap, such as
    castile or coconut oil
2 tablespoons vegetable glycerine
1 tablespoon water
4 slices dried loofah sponge, ½ inch
    thick

These are gentle scrubbing bars that are useful in cleaning your hands especially after a day of yard work or painting. You can also use them to help exfoliate your whole body. Do not use this soap to wash your face as it may be too harsh. I use a serrated bread knife to slice the dried loofah gourd.

Place the loofah slices on an oiled cookie sheet. In a double boiler gently heat the soap, glycerine, and water until you have a thick mixture and all the soap is melted. Spoon the melted soap inside your loofah slices and allow it to harden. Trim your soaps with a sharp knife.

To use: Enjoy as you would a loofah sponge or any scrubbing bar of soap. Avoid broken skin or sensitive areas.

Yield: 8 ounces, 3–4 bars of soap

Antiperspirants and Deodorants

*D*eodorant products are not exactly the most exciting to discuss, but they are an essential part of our daily routine. There is a wide variety of these products on the market, including sprays and creams in unscented and scented versions. They all share the same purpose: to keep you feeling fresh and clean and help control perspiration.

Perspiration helps regulate the body's temperature and releases salts and toxic substances from the body. Fresh perspiration is odorless; however, bacteria on the skin surface react with your perspiration to cause body odor. Body odor is not a pleasant smell, as anyone who has ridden a crowded bus or subway in the summer months can tell you. It can be cured and prevented by killing the odor-causing bacteria.

There are two main types of products that help prevent body odor—antiperspirants and deodorants. An antiperspirant has astringent properties in its ingredients that help reduce pore size and thus helps stop perspiration. Deodorants kill odor-causing bacteria. Many people prefer deodorants over antiperspirants, as they do not interfere with the body's natural release of moisture.

The products contained in this chapter require the general care and storage guidelines found on page 8.

Antiperspirant Spray

1 cup water
1½ teaspoons alum powder
    (U.S.P. grade)
¼ cup vodka

The key ingredient in this recipe is alum powder, which can be found at the drugstore. Make sure you use alum that is U.S.P. grade for cosmetic use. It is a powerful astringent, and combined with alcohol and water, it makes a very good natural antiperspirant.

Mix together all ingredients and stir well until the alum is dissolved. Pour into a spray bottle or a clean container with a tight-fitting lid.

To apply, spray on the body or use clean cotton pads.

Yield: 10 ounces

Natural Deodorant Cream

¼ cup vegetable shortening
1 tablespoon cornstarch
2 teaspoons baking soda
⅛ teaspoon tincture of benzoin
1 teaspoon fragrance (optional)

Cream deodorants are especially effective if you have very dry skin. My grandmother prefers to use scented creams on her delicate skin in place of deodorant sprays. Cream deodorants also work well in the winter months, when your skin tends to be a bit drier.

Blend all ingredients together into a smooth cream. Place in a clean jar with a tight-fitting lid.

To use: Rub a small amount of the cream under your arms.

Yield: 3 ounces

Botanical Deodorant

Witch hazel is a natural botanical astringent that makes a good base for a deodorant spray. Chlorophyll is another plant extract that has odor-absorbing properties. Adding a bit of glycerine makes this deodorant less drying than a pure alcohol spray, but it may feel a bit sticky at first. The stickiness goes away after the product has set for about a week.

Mix together all ingredients. Pour into a clean container or spray bottle.

To use: Spray under your arms or use clean cotton pads to apply.

Yield: 6 ounces

1 tablespoon glycerine
2 tablespoons vodka
½ cup witch hazel
½ teaspoon liquid chlorophyll
(see page 228)

Citrus Deodorant

If you have ever taken a fresh piece of citrus peel and rubbed your fingernail along it to release the essential oils, you cannot help but notice the fresh, clean scent. Lemons and other citrus fruits make perfect natural deodorants; their juice is mildly astringent and has antibacterial properties.

Mix together all ingredients in a ceramic bowl or glass jar. Let the mixture sit for one day, then strain off the liquid and discard the lemon zest. Pour into a clean container or spray bottle.

To use: Spray under your arms or use clean cotton pads to apply.

Yield: 4 ounces

1 tablespoon lemon zest
¼ cup water
¼ cup vodka
1 teaspoon liquid chlorophyll (see page 228)
3 drops bergamot oil (available at many health food stores)

Products for Men

*M*en are just as interested in caring for their bodies as women are. A man with clean skin and healthy hair can be very sexy. Looking good and feeling good about the way they look can also make men more confident. Today, men need more in their medicine cabinet than a deodorant stick and an aftershave splash; they need total skin, hair, and body-care products.

Most of the recipes in this book can be used by both men and women. Yet each sex does require its own unique products. Men shave their faces, and this creates a need for aftershaves, shaving creams, and lotions. Men also prefer bolder, spicier scents for many of their products. Share these recipes with your favorite man. Create the products together, or surprise him with his own unique line of cosmetics made by you. I like to make my husband aftershaves with his favorite scents and give them names that have a special meaning for us.

The products contained in this chapter require the general care and storage guidelines found on page 8.

SHAVING TIPS

In ancient times, the barbershop was an important part of daily life, a meeting place where information was exchanged and important decisions made. The barber was one of the most prominent members of the community. Alexander the Great and Julius Caesar were both regular customers, as they liked to keep their faces clean shaven. Native Americans shaved their faces, as did many of the early pioneers.

Today's shaving products have gotten a lot more sophisticated, but the shaving ritual continues as one of man's daily tasks. Here are some tips to follow when shaving.

- Always shave in the direction of hair growth. Shaving against the growth can cause ingrown hairs.

- Before shaving, soften the beard with warm water or a hot towel.

- Don't shave the same area over and over; this can be irritating and can damage new skin cell growth.

- Use a facial scrub once a week to remove dead skin and ingrown hairs.

- Rinse razor blades well after each use and allow to air-dry.

Bay Rum Aftershave

When my grandfathers and great-grandfathers would visit the local barbershop (the one with the candy cane–striped pole out front), bay rum was the aftershave the barber would slap on their faces. Today, it is still one of the most commonly used aftershaves. There are many versions of this old-fashioned skin tonic, but I like this recipe because it is so easy and has the same spicy, citrus scent I remember both of my grandfathers using.

½ cup vodka or witch hazel
2 tablespoons rum (Jamaican rum is preferred.)
2 dried bay leaves
¼ teaspoon whole allspice (found in the spice section at the grocery store)
1 cinnamon stick
Zest from one small orange (orange part only)

Mix together all ingredients. Pour into a clean jar with a tight-fitting lid. Place the jar in a dark, cool place for 2 weeks.

At the end of 2 weeks, strain off the liquid and pour into a clean container. Discard any zest and other remaining solids.

To use: Splash on the face after shaving.

Yield: 4 ounces

Soothing Aftershave

If your skin is very sensitive, or you have not shaved your face for a while, this is a good aftershave to try. Chamomile flowers, which look like tiny white daisies, are cooling and soothing to the face. Witch hazel, a well-known astringent, is especially comforting if you happen to cut yourself.

½ cup witch hazel
2 tablespoons vodka (optional)
2 tablespoons dried chamomile flowers (purchase at natural food stores or use chamomile tea)
⅛ teaspoon alum powder (optional)

Mix together all ingredients. Pour into a clean jar with a tight-fitting lid. Place the jar in a dark, cool place for 2 weeks.

At the end of 2 weeks, strain off the liquid and pour into a clean container. Discard any remaining solids. If you desire a stronger scent, add more chamomile flowers and let sit for another week, then strain as before.

To use: Splash on your face after shaving.

Yield: 4 ounces

Old West Aftershave

½ cup witch hazel

2 teaspoons apple cider vinegar

1 teaspoon dried or 3 teaspoons fresh sage leaves

⅛ teaspoon dried or ½ teaspoon fresh basil

¼ teaspoon whole allspice

⅛ teaspoon alum powder (optional)

Although most cowboys did not shave regularly, shaving was very much a part of the Wild West. We all remember the scenes from old westerns when the cowboys come to town for a hot bath and a shave. Old photos of such famous western legends as Doc Holliday and Wyatt Earp always show them clean shaven. This recipe is similar to one they would have used in those days.

Mix together all ingredients. Pour into a clean jar with a tight-fitting lid. Place the jar in a dark, cool place for 2 weeks.

At the end of 2 weeks, strain off the liquid, discard any solids, and pour into a clean container.

To use: Splash on your face after shaving.

Yield: 4 ounces

Roman Empire Aftershave

1 cup vodka or witch hazel

1½ teaspoons dried yarrow

1 tablespoon dried lavender flowers

1 tablespoon dried sage leaves

1 teaspoon dried mint

1 bay leaf

1 tablespoon glycerine (optional— use if you have dry skin)

Legend has it that in addition to being the extremely powerful leader of the Roman Empire, Julius Caesar was also very handsome and clean shaven. This aftershave recipe contains many herbs and scents commonly used during this period of history. Caesar may have splashed on a mixture similar to this when he visited Cleopatra!

Mix together all ingredients. Pour into a clean jar with a tight-fitting lid. Place the jar in a dark, cool place for 2 weeks.

At the end of 2 weeks, strain off the liquid and discard any solids; pour into a clean container.

After shaving, pour a small amount into your hands and pat on your face.

Note: If using fresh herbs, use 3 times the amount of dried herbs called for; for example, 1 tablespoon dried sage leaves equals 3 tablespoons fresh sage leaves.

Yield: 8 ounces

Vitalizing Skin Bracer

¼ cup vodka
¼ cup witch hazel
2 tablespoons distilled water
1 teaspoon camphor spirit

This skin bracer is used in much the same way as an aftershave. It contains less alcohol, so it is soothing and less drying to sensitive skin. Camphor spirit, from trees that grow in Java, China, and Brazil, gives a cool feeling to the skin and can be very exhilarating. (It is important to use camphor that says U.S.P. grade on the label—this means it is intended for cosmetic use.)

Mix together all ingredients. The mixture may seem cloudy at first, but it will clear after a few minutes. Pour into a clean container with a lid. Splash on the skin after shaving.

Yield: 6 ounces

Electric Pre-shave

½ cup vodka or witch hazel
2 tablespoons distilled water
1 tablespoon glycerine
½ teaspoon camphor spirit

When using an electric razor it's a good idea to use a pre-shave lotion to help the hairs stand up straight for a closer shave. Wash your face before applying the lotion, and always shave in the direction of hair growth. This recipe contains glycerine to make it less drying, and camphor to soothe and cool the skin.

Mix together all the ingredients. Pour into a clean container with a lid.

After washing your face, rub a small amount on your face and beard before shaving.

Yield: 6 ounces

Basic Shaving Cream

¼ cup stearic acid powder
1 cup hot water
1 teaspoon borax
2 tablespoons grated soap

The purpose of a good shaving cream is to help "set up" the beard, to facilitate razor glide, and to help the skin hold in the warm water that has been applied prior to smoothing on the shaving cream. This is a recipe my husband enjoys using because it is a mild and unscented cream.

In a double boiler on the stove top, melt the stearic acid powder until it is a clear liquid.

Mix together the hot water, borax, and soap, and stir until the borax and soap are completely dissolved. Pour the soap solution in a blender and turn on for about 1 minute, blending on low speed. Slowly pour the melted stearic acid liquid into the soap solution. Blend on high until a smooth cream has formed.

Pour into a clean, open container and allow to cool completely. When cool, stir the cream and put into a container with a tight-fitting lid or cover with plastic wrap.

To use: Soften your beard with warm water and then smooth the shaving cream over your face. Use a sharp, clean razor.

Note: You may need to give this cream a good stirring from time to time if it's been sitting on a shelf, but if you are using it every day this will probably not be necessary.

Yield: 8 ounces

CLEANSING FACIAL SCRUBS

One advantage of shaving (although my husband will argue that there are none) is that it exfoliates, that is, removes dead skin cells from the face. Good skin care for men also includes using a face scrub once a week. Make sure you choose a scrub that is suitable for the face — small, fine, well-rounded grains work best (no pumice scrubs, please). Any of the cleansing scrubs in this book work well for both men and women. For men I would suggest the following scrubs: cornmeal, ground dried orange and lime peel, and ground sunflower seeds (unsalted and without the shell).

Take a teaspoon of one of the above scrubs and mix together with water, or soap and water, to form a smooth paste.

Massage the paste gently into your skin for about 3 to 5 minutes, and rinse well with tepid water.

Almond Oil Shaving Cream

Adding almond oil to the basic shaving cream in the previous recipe will make a richer, more moisturizing cream. If you are prone to dry skin, I would suggest using this recipe. If your skin is flaking or chapped, you may even want to add a little extra oil.

¼ cup stearic acid powder
2 tablespoons almond oil (or any other light oil)
1 cup hot water
1 teaspoon borax
2 tablespoons grated soap

In a double boiler on the stove top, melt the stearic acid powder and oil until it is a clear liquid.

Mix together the hot water, borax, and soap, and stir until the borax and soap are completely dissolved. Pour the soap solution in a blender and blend well for about 1 minute. Slowly pour the melted stearic acid mixture into the soap solution. Blend on high until a smooth cream has formed.

Pour into a clean container and allow to cool completely.

To use: Soften your beard with warm water and then smooth the shaving cream over your face. Use a sharp, clean razor.

Yield: 8 ounces

Invigorating Foot Rub

This is a nice treat after a long day on your feet. It is twice as much fun to have someone give you a foot rub — and, of course, to return the favor! The effective ingredients in this recipe are the vinegar and camphor oil. Because they are mildly astringent and cooling, they assist in stimulating and energizing your feet.

2 tablespoons sunflower oil (or any light oil)
½ teaspoon vinegar
½ teaspoon alum powder (U.S.P. grade)
¼ teaspoon camphor oil

Mix together all ingredients and stir well. Pour into a clean container with a tight-fitting lid. Store in a cool, dark place.

To use: Pour a small amount into your palm and slowly massage into your feet. Repeat until your tired feet feel alive and refreshed. Put your feet up and read a good magazine for at least 15 minutes.

Yield: 2 ounces, 1 foot rub

Athlete's-Foot Cure

Geranium oil, found in many health food stores, is an excellent cure for athlete's foot because it has germ- and bacteria-killing properties. Athlete's-foot germs thrive in warm, damp environments, so always keep your feet clean and dry, especially between the toes, where moisture can get trapped. If you should get athlete's foot—an itchy foot rash, blisters, and flaky skin—here are two cures to try, both using geranium oil.

FOOT BATH

FOOT BATH:

Fill a shallow tub or sink with warm water. Add the salt and geranium oil; stir to dissolve the salt.

Soak your feet for 20 minutes. Dry well, especially between the toes, and follow with a good moisturizer or foot powder.

Warm water
½ cup salt
5 drops geranium oil

FOOT MASSAGE OIL

1 tablespoon light oil
10 drops geranium oil

Yield: 1 treatment

FOOT MASSAGE OIL:

Mix together the two oils. Massage each foot for at least 5 minutes.

Yield: ½ ounce, 1 treatment

Pumice Hand Scrub

1¼ cups soap flakes
2 tablespoons borax
1 tablespoon powdered pumice or
 fine sand

If your hands are really dirty and grimy after working on the car or painting the house, this scrub will get them really clean. An olive oil rinse will also work to remove the last stubborn bits of grime and keep your hands in good condition.

Mix together all the ingredients. Place in a clean container with a tight-fitting lid.

To use: Scoop out a small amount and mix with warm water to form a lather and clean the hands. Rinse thoroughly with warm water.

Note: You can make your own powdered pumice by smashing a bit of pumice stone with a hammer. Place the stone in a thick plastic bag to keep it clean and all the small pieces together. Pound until the pumice is the size of fine sand or table salt.

Yield: 12 ounces

Avocado Oil Hair Pack

½ avocado, mashed (If you have
 long hair, you may need a whole
 avocado.)
1 teaspoon avocado oil (optional, for
 very dry hair)

Many men today are often concerned with their hair growth — or lack thereof. Avocados make an effective hair-conditioning pack because they are rich in vitamins A, D, and E — all necessary for healthy hair. I have read claims that the oil is easily absorbed into the scalp, stimulating new hair growth. If you have a very dry scalp, you may want to add the teaspoon of avocado oil.

Massage the mashed avocado into your hair and scalp. Wrap your hair in plastic wrap or use a plastic shower cap; leave the conditioner on your hair for 15 minutes. Shampoo your hair as usual and rinse well.

Yield: 1 treatment

Horseradish Hair Treatment

Horseradish has a hot, refreshing taste and adds zip to a meal when used as a condiment. It also makes a wonderful hair treatment. A member of the cabbage family, these roots increase blood flow to the skin, a process that prevents hair loss. It is best to use fresh roots, available at many grocery stores. The yogurt is added to give the treatment a smoother consistency.

¼ cup freshly grated horseradish root
¼ cup plain yogurt

Mix together the horseradish and yogurt to form a smooth paste. Massage this mixture into your hair and scalp. Wrap your hair in plastic wrap or use a plastic shower cap; leave the conditioner on your hair for 15 minutes. Shampoo your hair as usual and rinse well.

Note: If you cannot find fresh horseradish, you may use bottled horseradish instead.

Yield: 1 treatment

Moustache Wax

This wax will help keep your moustache in place and looking well groomed. Castor oil helps to strengthen the hair by coating it and forming a tough, shiny, protective covering. (You can also use this recipe to tame unruly eyebrows.)

2 teaspoons grated beeswax
1 teaspoon castor oil

Mix together the beeswax and castor oil in a heat-resistant container. Heat the mixture gently in the microwave on High, or on the stove top in a water bath until the beeswax is melted, stirring.

Pour into a clean container and allow to cool until solid. Rub your finger over the cool wax and apply sparingly to your moustache or eyebrows.

Yield: ½ ounce

Crew-Cut Oil

2 teaspoons coconut oil
1 teaspoon castor oil

You don't need to sport a crew cut to use this hair dressing, but it does work particularly well on short hair. It also works wonders on black hair to keep it looking healthy and shiny. The coconut oil and castor oil protect and strengthen the hair and help prevent breakage.

Warm the coconut oil—this can be done in the microwave on High or on the stove top—until it is melted. Add the castor oil, stirring until well mixed. Pour into a clean container and allow to cool.

To use: Rub a small amount through your hair. Be careful to use sparingly or your hair may appear greasy.

Yield: 1 ounce

Products for Children

Children's bath products vary from adult products in that young people have finer hair, sensitive skin, and more delicate noses. Strong scents and ingredients are not appropriate for immature systems. Instead, lightly scented products containing pure, natural ingredients are best for cleaning and moisturizing skin and hair. It is important to keep children's skin clean, dry, and fresh. Doing this will greatly reduce the risk of skin problems or rashes that some children can develop.

Bathing should also be fun. If you make it something your child wants to do, you help your children develop good health habits. My girls know better than to go to bed with dirty skin and hair. Making bath time enjoyable seems to take some of the chore out of it. I have always encouraged them to be creative in the bath, and if this means hauling out all the cooking tools for a bathtub restaurant or tinting the water green, we have done it!

Many of the recipes in this section are easy to create. Children can make them along with their parents, although very young children may need more help. They also make wonderful presents for birthdays and holidays. Mix up a batch of Scented Play Dough, page 299, or Fantasy Face Paints, page 298, to take to a friend's house.

Children's bath products should be stored in clean, non-breakable containers. Plastic seems to work best. It is always a good idea to keep any cosmetic product, even natural ones, where children cannot get into them. Something that smells good is often a temptation and could upset a small stomach if ingested.

Childhood is all about enjoying yourself and having fun. I always tell my daughters that life is meant to be lived and their job is to be the best at it!

Baby Powder

1 cup cornstarch
½ teaspoon light oil (almond, apricot kernel, mineral)
¼ teaspoon liquid chlorophyll
2–3 drops lavender oil

This is a lovely, rich powder for all ages, but it's ideal for keeping infants comfortable. Australian mothers often put a drop or two of lavender oil in their babies' baths—the oil and cornstarch keep them dry and happy. Most commercial baby powders are pure talc with added fragrance, but many mothers choose not to use talc products around their children. (Talc can be a lung irritant if breathed over a period of time.) For a variation, try using rose or jasmine oil in place of the lavender oil.

There are two methods to choose from in mixing this powder, using a blender or a sealable container.

BLENDER METHOD:

Place the cornstarch in the blender, and blend on low. With the blender still running, slowly add the oil, chlorophyll, and lavender oil, one at a time. When well mixed, pour into a clean container.

You may apply with a shaker-type container, or use a pretty jar with a powder puff.

CONTAINER METHOD:

Place the cornstarch in a resealable jar, plastic bag, or container. Add the oil, chlorophyll, and lavender oil. Seal the container and shake gently until the powder is well mixed and the oils and chlorophyll are dispersed.

You may apply with a shaker-type container, or use a pretty jar with a powder puff.

Yield: 8 ounces

Baby Oil

Many of the commercial baby oils on the market today are simply mineral oil with a scent. It is easy to make your own using pure, light, natural oils. Apricot kernel oil is made from the oil-rich nut inside the fruit's seed or pit and can be found at many natural food stores. I like to make this recipe unscented, but if you prefer a subtle fragrance, I would suggest using the mild essential oil of sweet orange, chamomile, or lavender—but only a drop or two.

¼ cup apricot kernel oil
1 tablespoon light sesame oil
½ tablespoon wheat germ oil
1–2 drops essential oil of sweet orange, chamomile, or lavender (optional)

Stir together all ingredients and pour into a clean, dry container with a tight-fitting lid.

To use: Massage a small amount into warm or damp skin. Store in a cool, dark, dry location.

Yield: 3 ounces

BABY MASSAGE

The ancient art of baby massage has gained renewed interest. Once regarded as an essential skill of motherhood passed down from mother to daughter, this activity had been all but lost in our society until recently. There are now classes for new mothers, books, and even videos on the art of baby massage. It is believed that by gently massaging your baby's body, he or she will grow stronger, sleep better, eat more, and even gain relief from colic. It also encourages bonding and acts as a form of communication between new parents and their baby.

Because babies are so new to the world and their sense of smell extremely sensitive, I would not use scented oil when massaging a baby less than 12 months of age. Pure, sweet almond oil works well and is gentle enough for a newborn.

(continued)

I used to massage my babies after bathing them and before putting them to bed at night. You should choose a time that is relaxing and enjoyable for both of you. Here are the basic steps I followed:

1. Sit with your baby on your lap or place your baby on a soft mat in front of you. It is important that you are both in a comfortable position.

2. With your baby facing you, place your hands on his or her hips, and slide your hand up to the shoulders, then down the sides of his or her body. Repeat several times.

3. Massage your baby's stomach, gently stroking it in a circular motion.

4. Stroke the back of your baby's hands and then the palms. Gently squeeze each finger and repeat with the other hand.

5. Massage the arms. Holding his or her hand in yours, stroke in a flowing motion from the shoulder to the wrist.

6. Massage the legs. Hold his or her foot in your hand and stroke each leg from the thigh to the ankle. Repeat several times. Squeeze and rotate each toe and massage the foot.

7. Turn your baby over and massage his or her back. Use calm, gentle strokes. Slow, light strokes are very soothing to your baby.

You and your baby will soon be looking forward to this special time of comfort and relaxation. Enjoy!

Coconut Baby Oil

Coconut oil is used to make adult skin and hair care products and is also mild enough for children's products. This is a rich tropical recipe that is perfect for use in massage or after bath. I like to use it on my daughters' feet in the summer to keep them soft and smooth after a day of running around barefoot.

2 tablespoons coconut oil
½ tablespoon grated cocoa butter
2 tablespoons castor oil

In a heat-resistant container mix together all the ingredients. Heat gently in the microwave or in a water bath until the coconut oil and cocoa butter are melted. Stir well and let the mixture cool completely. Spoon into a clean container.

To use: Massage a small amount into warm skin after bathing.

Yield: 2 ounces

Diaper Cream

Today, with the use of washing machines and disposable diapers, diaper rash is no longer the common baby rash it once was. Babies' bottoms are kept drier, and they are getting changed more often. This keeps their delicate skin dry and comfortable and gives it a chance to breathe. If your little one's delicate bum does happen to break out, this old-fashioned cure has stood the test of time. It contains liquid lecithin, a substance extracted from soybeans and used for ages as an excellent moisturizer and diaper ointment. It protects baby's sensitive skin and keeps it dry. It should be applied once a day. For extreme cases, use this cream every time you change your baby's diaper.

2 tablespoons soy lecithin
1 teaspoon coconut oil
1 teaspoon apricot kernel oil
¼ teaspoon vitamin E oil
½ cup distilled water

Mix together the lecithin, coconut oil, apricot kernel oil, and vitamin E oil. Heat this mixture gently until the coconut oil is liquefied. Gently heat the distilled water until it is roughly the same temperature as the oil mixture. Pour the lecithin mixture into a blender and start stirring. Slowly add the warm water and blend on High until the mixture is thick and creamy. Pour the cream into a clean container and allow it to cool completely, stirring occasionally.

To use: Apply a small amount onto your baby's clean bottom before diapering.

Note: You can adjust this cream's consistency by adding more or less water to the recipe.

Yield: 6 ounces

New Baby Bath

¼ cup dry nonfat milk powder
¼ cup dry buttermilk powder
1 tablespoon cornstarch

This is a gentle milk bath that will leave your baby's tender skin soft and silky. Milk is rich in fat and lactic acid, and both help soften and hydrate the skin. Prepare an extra portion of this treatment for yourself because everyone can use a rich, relaxing natural bath—especially new parents!

Mix together all the ingredients and pour into a clean container or resealable plastic bag.

To use: Pour ¼ cup of the bath powder into a full tub or 1 tablespoon into a small baby bathtub.

Yield: 4 ounces, enough for 2 full baths

Honey Bee Bath

Honey is one of my favorite natural beauty ingredients because it is so versatile and offers amazing results. It is a natural humectant, which means it has the ability to attract and retain moisture. This recipe makes a wonderful bath for dry, sensitive skin and is gentle enough for children of all ages. You can use any variety of honey in this sweet recipe; I like to use clover or orange blossom varieties.

1 cup water
½ cup honey
½ cup mild liquid soap

Mix together all the ingredients and pour into a clean bottle with a tight-fitting stopper or lid.

To use: Gently shake the bottle to reblend and pour ¼ cup into the bath under the running water.

Yield: 16 ounces, enough for 8 baths

Fresh Strawberry Bath

This is a fruit-scented bath that is perfect for dry, delicate skin. It makes the bathwater a creamy shade of pink and contains two natural emollients—fresh cream and castor oil. Castor oil has been used for years as a health tonic. It comes from the seeds of the castor plant. This oil is used in many bath products because it easily disperses through the bathwater rather than floating on top as other oils do.

½ cup fresh strawberries (or frozen)
½ cup heavy cream
2 cups water
1 tablespoon castor oil

Place all of the ingredients into a blender and process on High until you have a smooth, creamy liquid. You may strain this mixture if you like.

To use: Pour the strawberry mixture into a warm bath and stir well.

Yield: 24 ounces, enough for 1 bath

Bubbles, Bubbles, Bubbles

2 cups liquid soap
6 cups water
¾ cup light corn syrup

Children of all ages love a good old-fashioned bubble bath. This recipe does double duty as it can be used in the bath and out. You can use this mixture to blow superbubbles for extra bathtime fun. Fashion your own bubble wand out of a pipe cleaner or look around the house for unique bubble gadgets such as plastic berry baskets, vented spatulas, or cheese graters.

Mix together all ingredients and let sit for at least 4 hours. Pour into a clean container with a tight-fitting lid.

To use: Pour ½ cup into the bath under running water. For bubbles, pour solution into a plastic dish and use bubble wands to blow bubbles into the air.

Yield: 64 ounces

HAVE FUN!

Encourage creativity when it comes to cleaning up. Here are a few ideas to get you started:

- **Grooming chart:** Draw or cut out pictures from magazines of people taking care of themselves. Glue these on a chart or calendar and give your children a star every time they brush their teeth, wash their face, or take a bath.

- **Music:** Play upbeat songs, nature sounds, or classical tunes to create or enhance the mood of your bathroom.

- **Bath toys:** Make your own washcloth puppets from terry cloth, create funny sponge shapes, or make bath puzzles by cutting up plastic place mats (they will stick to wet shower walls).

- **Bubbles:** The bath is the perfect place to blow bubbles (see recipe above).

Sweet Dreams Bath

This bath is like a warm hug at the end of a busy day. It contains chamomile and oatmeal, both of which are soothing and calming to young bodies. After the bath let your child snuggle into his or her bed while you read aloud a favorite book.

½ cup dried chamomile or chamomile tea
2 cups oatmeal
¼ cup cornstarch

Place all the ingredients inside a food processor or blender. Grind until you have a smooth, fine powder, which should have the consistency of whole-grain flour. Pour into a clean, airtight container or use a resealable plastic bag.

To use: Pour ½ cup into your bath as you fill the tub.

Yield: 16 ounces, enough for 4 baths

Tutti-Frutti Lip Gloss

Mix up batches of these fruit-flavored lip glosses to tuck inside backpacks, coat pockets, and bedside drawers. Little lips need protection, especially during the winter months. I like to use fruit-flavored oils from the grocery store, the same ones used in baking. You may also use fruit-flavored powdered juice mixes.

1 teaspoon coconut oil
1 teaspoon vegetable shortening
2 drops fruit-flavored oil or ⅛ teaspoon fruit-flavored drink mix

Mix together the coconut oil and shortening and stir well until smooth and creamy. Add the flavored oil. Stir well and spoon into a clean small jar or lip gloss container.

To use: Spread on lips.

Yield: ½ ounce

Marie's Glitter Gloss

2 teaspoons grated beeswax
2 tablespoons light oil such as
    almond
1 teaspoon honey
⅛ teaspoon fine glitter

My daughter Marie loves anything glittery, especially when it comes to bath and body products. This sweet-tasting lip gloss is fun to wear for a special day out shopping or having fun with friends. It can also be used as body glitter, to add a hint of glamour to cheeks and shoulders. Shop for fine glitter at better craft stores and make sure it is non-toxic.

Put the beeswax, oil, and honey in a heat-resistant container and heat gently in the microwave or water bath until the beeswax is melted. Add glitter and stir well. Pour the mixture into a small jar or lip gloss container and let cool completely.

To use: Spread on lips; if using as a body gloss, avoid the eye area.

Yield: 1½ ounces

Fantasy Face Paints

1 teaspoon cornstarch
1 teaspoon water
½ teaspoon cold cream (see Basic
    Cold Cream recipe on page 63)
1–2 drops food coloring

Children love to play dress up and imagine they are princesses, pirates, frogs, bears, and all sort of wonderful characters. They can use this gentle face paint made from cold cream and cornstarch to paint their faces and bodies. I use food coloring from the grocery store for the color, but you may also experiment with fresh berry juices and plant dyes to tint your face paints—just be sure they are safe for cosmetic use. You will need to mix up a batch for each color or double the recipe and divide it into small bowls before adding your color.

Mix together the cornstarch, water, and cold cream and stir well until smooth. Add food coloring 1 drop at a time and mix until you are pleased with the shade. Spoon into a small jar or bowl. I have found reusable plastic paint palettes from art stores are good containers for your homemade paints.

To use: Paint the skin in any design you desire using a small brush, cotton swab, or a clean fingertip. Clean off your designs with more cold cream and warm water.

Yield: ½ ounce

Scented Play Dough

Mix up a batch of this scented dough to have on hand when the kids need a quiet activity or you have children visiting. I like to use lavender oil to scent my dough, but other safe scents to use would be rose, vanilla, orange, peach, or coconut. Working and molding the scented mixture is a creative and calming activity. This recipe also makes a fun birthday gift for a special child—fill a bright plastic tub with cookie cutters, miniature kitchen gadgets, a small rolling pin, and a batch of scented play dough!

1 cup flour
½ cup salt
1 cup water (may be tinted with food coloring)
1 tablespoon sunflower oil
2 teaspoons cream of tartar
2–3 drops scented oil

Mix together the flour, salt, water, oil, and cream of tartar in a medium-size saucepan. Cook the mixture over medium heat until it begins to bubble. Remove the pan from the heat and stir in the scented oil. Place the dough on a lightly floured board and knead for 3 to 5 minutes until smooth. Store in an airtight container.

To use: Shape your dough into anything you desire. Store any leftover dough in a clean airtight container or resealable plastic bag. If left uncovered and allowed to air-dry, your designs will dry out and harden.

Yield: 8 ounces

Glossary of Terms

Acid: An acid can be liquid, solid, or gas. It is a substance that contains hydrogen and reacts with metals to form salts and water. You can usually tell an acid by its pH level, which is below 7. Examples of common acids are citric acid (lemon juice), acetic acid (vinegar), and tannic acid (found in tea).

Alcohol: A colorless, volatile liquid obtained by distillation and fermentation of carbohydrates (grain, molasses, potatoes). Alcohol is antiseptic and cooling but is also very drying to the hair and skin; thus care should be taken not to use too much.

Anhydrous: If a substance is anhydrous, it does not contain water.

Antiperspirant: A product that inhibits or prevents perspiration.

Antiseptic: It stops the growth of bacteria and helps to control infection by inhibiting germs.

Azulene: An anti-inflammatory agent extracted from chamomile and yarrow flowers. Azulene is known for its skin-soothing qualities.

Collagen: Collagen is the substance that gives your skin elasticity, or the ability to stretch. It is found in the inner layer of the skin, or dermis.

Combination skin: When you have both dry and oily areas. This is the most common skin type.

Cosmetic: The official Federal Drug Act definition of cosmetics, which has not changed since 1938, is: (1) articles intended to be rubbed, poured, sprinkled, or sprayed on, introduced into, or otherwise applied to the human body or any part thereof for cleansing, beautifying, promoting attractiveness, or altering the appearance, and (2) articles intended for use as a component of any such articles.

Dermis: The inner layer of the skin. The dermis is protected by the epidermis and is made up of tissues, muscles, and nerves. Collagen is found in the dermis layer.

Dry skin: If your skin feels tight after washing and has a tendency to flake, your pores are small, and your skin is thin, you have dry skin.

Emollient: A thick, creamy material used to soothe or soften the skin. Emollients are usually made from oil, water, and wax.

Emulsifier: A material that binds two different materials together. An example of this would be using beeswax when making cold cream to bind together the oil and water and keep them from separating.

Epidermis: The surface layer of the skin. The epidermis is where new cells are constantly being formed.

Exfoliation: Removal of dead skin cells and surface dirt. A very important step in proper skin care, as removing dead skin cells allows the skin to function more efficiently and to absorb more moisture.

Facial: A total treatment for the face that consists of deep cleansing, conditioning, and moisturizing of the skin.

Halitosis: Bad breath.

Herb: A plant or plant part valued for its medicinal, savory, or aromatic qualities. For example, chamomile is very soothing to the skin, peppermint has a scent that is extremely refreshing, and geranium oil kills bacteria.

Humectant: A substance that holds the moisture in a product or on the skin. Honey is a wonderful natural humectant. Glycerine is the most popular humectant used in cosmetic products.

Infusion: A mixture of herbs and water that is soaked together for a period of time. When you make tea, you are making an infusion.

Keratin: Sulfur-containing fibrous proteins that form the chemical basis of horny epidermal tissues such as hair and nails.

Mucilage: A gelatinous substance that contains protein and polysaccharides (sugars) and is similar to plant gums.

Natural: This term is loosely used and no one seems to agree on its definition in regard to cosmetics. The FDA is currently trying to come up with an official definition. I think of natural as not containing any man-made ingredients. Natural to me means "as found in nature." Some feel that natural means no chemicals—but chemicals are natural. Everything in our world is made up of chemical elements.

Normal skin: Clear, firm skin with few blemishes; not dry or oily.

Oily skin: If your face feels a little greasy, with a shine that does not go away, enlarged pores, and no lines, you have oily skin.

Organic: A substance that is, or once was, living. In chemistry, organic means "containing a carbon atom."

pH (potential hydrogen): The degree of acidity or alkalinity of a substance is its pH. A neutral pH is 7 (the pH of water and blood), a pH below 7 is considered acidic, and a pH above 7 is alkaline. For example, lemon juice has a pH of 3, while baking soda has a pH of 9. If you wish to test the pH of a product, you can do so very easily with litmus paper, which can be purchased at many drug-stores. Follow the directions on the package. Typically, orange to pink indicates an acid, and green to purple an alkaline.

Sebum: An oil secreted by the skin.

Ultraviolet light: The invisible light rays that penetrate the epidermis and have been proven to cause premature aging and skin cancer.

U.S.P.: You will see this labeling on many products such as lanolin, camphor, glycerine, and alum powder. U.S.P. stands for United States Pharmacopeia and means that the product meets the standards for use set out by the United States Pharmaceutical Board.

Water bath: A water bath is a method for heating ingredients when making cosmetics. Simply place a container with the ingredients into a pan with one to two inches of water already in it. It's similar to a double boiler, as it protects ingredients from direct heat. Also known as a *bain marie.*

Index

acids, neutralizing, 16
acne, 109
   Strawberry Acne mask, 108
After-Bath Splash, 222
aftershaves, 15, 275
   Bay Rum, 277
   Old West, 278
   Roman Empire, 278–79
   Soothing, 277
age, and skin type, 58, 61
alcohol, 47
   in fragrances, 214
   for massage, 166
   natural, 24
alkanet root, 120
allergies and sensitivities, 8
Alligator Pear Lotion, 80–81
Allover Nighttime Lotion,
   79–80
All-Purpose Honey Cleanser,
   34
Almond
   Cleansing Scrub, 38
   and Cocoa Butter Lip Gloss,
    116
   Coconut-Almond Lip Gloss,
    117

Almond oil, 8, 15, 76
   for baby massage, 291
   Hair Gel, 192
   Lotion, 67–68
   Powder, 231
   Shaving Cream, 282
aloe vera, 15
   Lip Gloss, 116
   in shampoo, 175
   Gel, Floral, 77
   Lotion, Cooling, 78
alum (aluminum sulfate), 15
alum powder, 270
ambergris, 214
Amorous Massage Oil, 161
antibacterial agents, 23
   honey, 108
anti-itch treatment, aspirin as, 16
antimicrobials, 122
antioxidants, 19, 56
   lecithin, 99
   vitamin C, 23, 54
antiperspirants, 269–71
   Antiperspirant Spray, 270
antiseptic, 15
   aspirin, 16
   honey, 99

   lavender oil, 57
   tincture of benzoin, 23
   zinc oxide, 26
apple cider vinegar
   hair rinse, 184
Apple Juice Astringent, 49
Apricot Facial Mask, 96
apricot kernel oil (persic oil), 15,
   24
   in baby oil, 291
Apricot Kernel Scrub, 41
aromatherapy, 129, 131, 159–68
aromatherapy shops, 18
aromatic oils, 214, 216
arrowroot, 246
   Cleansing Jelly, 35
aspirin (salicylic acid), 16, 108
astringents, 15, 47, 48–49
   Apple Juice, 49
   Basic, 48
   cucumber, 66
   cucumber juice, 51
   grapefruit, 36
   lemon juice, 33
   for Sensitive Skin, 48
   Strawberry Leaf, 49
   zinc oxide, 26

Athlete's-Foot Cure, 283
Attar of Roses, 223
Australian Frangipani Lotion,
    68–69
Australian Lanolin Cream, 70–71
avocado oil, 16, 73
    Hair Pack, 284
avocado pits, 27
avocados, 13, 16, 80
    as mask, 106
Avocado-Stone Scrub, 40–41
Azulene, 83

B vitamins, 16, 101, 104, 132
baby massage, 291–92
Baby Oil, 291
    Coconut, 293
Baby Powder, 290
bacteria, 109, 227, 269
    in mouth, 241, 242, 245
bad breath, 241, 242
baking soda (sodium
        bicarbonate), 13, 16
    hair rinse, 184
    tooth powder, 245–46
banana
    as mask, 106
Basic Astringent, 48
Basic Castile Soap, 255–56
Basic Cold Cream, 63–64
Basic Hair Gel, 190–91
Basic Moisturizer, 71–72
Basic Shampoo A, 173
Basic Shampoo B, 173
Basic Shaving Cream, 280–81
basil, 162
    effects of, 130
    Shampoo Powder, 178
    in soap, 264
Bath Bombs, Fizzing, 135
bath environment, ultimate, 138
Bath Powder
    Scented, 229
    Simple, 228, 230

Bath Salts
    Colored, 132–33
    Foaming, 136
bath treatments/baths, 125–38
    After-Bath Splash, 222
    babies, 290, 294
    bubble bath, 133, 296
    children, 289, 290, 294–97
    Cleopatra Milk Bath, 128
    Colored Bath Salts, 132–33
    Fizzing Bath Bombs, 135
    Foaming Bath Salts, 136
    following dry brushing, 148
    herb baths, 129–30
    Honey Bee Bath, 295
    milk, 125, 128
    Morning Wake-up!, 126
    Mustard Bath, 136
    New Baby Bath, 294
    Northwest Pine Bath, 130–31
    Oatmeal Cookie Bath, 132
    Old-Fashioned Bubble Bath,
        133
    Pineapple Body Seltzer,
        126–27
    Relaxing Lavender Bath, 137
    Rose Floral Bath, 131
    Scrubbing Sacks, 134
    Super Muscle-Soothing Bath,
        129
    Sweet Dreams Bath, 297
    Vinegar-Herb Bath, 127–28
    water temperature, 125, 138
Bay Rum Aftershave, 277
beauty basics, 4
    see also natural beauty
Beauty Mayo, 94
Beauty Queen Mask, 99
beauty tools
    from nature, 26–28
beauty treatments, 3, 4, 5
    see also ingredients; natural
        beauty products
Beauty Water, 57

bee supply stores, 14, 16
beef fat, 251
beer, 15, 16
    Body and Bounce Beer
        Shampoo, 175
    hair rinse, 184
    Tucson Jojoba Oil and Beer
        Conditioner, 182
beeswax, 14, 16
    Lipsticks, 119–20
beetroots, 263
Bentonite, 100
bergamot
    effects of, 130
    scent, 168
beta-carotene, 96
birth control pills, 7
blender/food processor, 12
blue cornmeal, 14
Body and Bounce Beer Shampoo,
    175
body brushes, 144
Body Butter, 73–74
body glitter
    Marie's Glitter Gloss, 298
Body Lotion, Mint, 84–85
Body Mask
    Green Goddess, 151
    Sea Mud, 145–46
Body Massage, English Ivy,
    149–50
body odor, 227, 235, 269
Body Polish, Tropical, 147
body treatments, 141–55
    English Ivy Body Massage,
        149–50
    Green Goddess Body Mask,
        151
    Herbal Body Wrap, 145
    Loofah Body Polish, 152
    Mehndi-Henna Tattoos,
        152–53
    Raw Sugar Scrub, 143
    Salt Rub, 142

Sea Mud Body Mask, 145–46
seawater, 146
Sunburn Soothers, 155
Tropical Body Polish, 147
Yogurt Body Treatment, 147
Body Wrap, Herbal, 145
borax (sodium tetraborate), 17
Botanical Deodorant, 271
bottles/pitchers, 13, 252
bowls, 12, 13
breathing, 168
Brewer's Yeast Mask, 104
Brilliantine, 193
bromelain, 107, 126, 206
Bubble Bath, Old-Fashioned,
133
Bubbles, Bubbles, Bubbles,
296

calcium, 106
calendula flowers, 77
California Cold Cream, 65–66
camphor, 164
camphor spirit, 279
candy thermometers, 252
cantaloupe, hair conditioner,
181
carbon dioxide, 16
Caribbean Rum Conditioner,
183
Carmen Miranda Fruit Powder,
236
carmine, 120
carrageenan, 85
carrots, 96
Fresh Carrot Mask, 108
castile soap, 13, 17, 262
Basic, 255–56
castor oil, 17, 37, 76, 193, 214,
285
Lip Balm, 119
Nail Rub, 208
chamomile, 18, 78, 162
in bath, 197

effects of, 130
in hair-care products, 174, 178,
185
Skin Freshener, 53–54
in soap, 264
chamomile flowers
in aftershave, 277
Champagne Hair Gel, 193
Chapped Lip Cure, 121
chickpeas, 102
children, products for, 289–99
Baby Oil, 291
Baby Powder, 290
baths, 294–97
Bubbles, Bubbles, Bubbles, 296
Coconut Baby Oil, 293
Diaper Cream, 293–94
Fantasy Face Paints, 298–99
Fresh Srawberry Bath, 295
fun in cleaning up, 296
Honey Bee Bath, 295
Marie's Glitter Gloss, 298
New Baby Bath, 294
Scented Play Dough, 299
Sweet Dreams Bath, 297
Tutti-Frutti Lip Glow, 297
China clay, 100
chlorophyll, 17, 228, 263, 271
Chocolate Lip Gloss, 3, 118
chromium, 109
cinnamon
hair rinse, 185
Powder, Cooling, 238
scent, 161
citric acid, 20, 36
citronella, 213
Citrus
Deodorant, 271
Dry Perfume, 222
Freshener, 55
fruits, 20
Massage Oil, 163
peeler and zester, 11
scents, 176

civet, 214
clay, 92
Natural Clay Masks, 99–100
cleansers, 23, 29–37
All-Purpose Honey, 34
Arrowroot Cleansing Jelly,
35
Cleansing Milk, 33
Country Fresh Dairy, 37
Empress Josephine's, 34
Gentle Eye Makeup Remover,
37
Grapefruit, 36
Oatmeal, 33
Olive Oil Cleansing Lotion,
35
Strawberry, 36
see also scrubs
Cleansing Milk, 33
Cleopatra, 5, 125, 224
Milk Bath, 128
scents, 213
Cloud Nine Powder, 237
Clove Mouthwash, 243
clove oil, 166
cocoa butter, 13, 17, 19, 73, 82
Almond and, Lip Gloss, 116
Cocoa Cuticle Cream, 204
Coconut
-Almond Lip Gloss, 117
Baby Oil, 293
Cloud Cream, 72–73
Flavored, Lip Gloss, 117
coconut oil, 14, 17, 70, 72, 73,
82
Soap, 256–57
coffee grinder, 12
Cold Cream
Basic, 62, 63–64
California, 65–66
Cucumber, 66–67
Original Greek, 64–65
Soap, 258–59
cold sores, 122

Cologne, 18, 214
    Eau de, 217
    Irresistible Rose, 218
    Orchid Isle, 219
    Summer Garden, 220
    Victoria Handkerchief, 218
color, 168
    in bath environment, 138
Colored Bath Salts, 132–33
colored soap, 263
combination skin (type), 58, 61
commercial products, 5, 8, 214
Cooling Aloe Lotion, 78
Cooling Cinnamon Powder, 238
Cooling Cucumber Toner, 51
Cooling Eye Gel, 111
Cooling Massage Spirits, 165
Corn Flour Lotion, 73
cornmeal
    dry shampoo, 177
    scrub, 281
cornstarch (corn flour), 13, 18,
        35, 73
    in powders, 227
cosmetics, 4–5
    flowers in, 18
    making one's own, 5
cotton, 27
cotton washcloth, 144
Country Fresh Dairy Cleanser, 37
Country Garden Facial Mask, 96
creams, 23, 61–87
    Australian Lanolin, 70–71
    Basic Cold Cream, 63–64
    Body Butter, 73–74
    California Cold Cream, 65–66
    Coconut Cloud, 72–73
    Cucumber Cold Cream, 66–67
    cuticle, 202, 204
    Diaper Cream, 293–94
    Firming Neck, 82
    Original Greek Cold Cream,
        64–65
    Papaya, 75

Stretch Mark, 86
Super Eye, 81
Tropical Eye, 82–83
Crew-Cut Oil, 286
crow's feet, 110
Cucumber
    Cold Cream, 66–67
    Cooling Cucumber Toner, 51
    as mask, 106
cucumber juice, 66
cuticles, 201, 202
    Cocoa Cuticle Cream, 204
    creams, 202, 204
    Jojoba Nail and Cuticle Oil,
        204
    Pineapple Cuticle Softener, 206

dairy products, 32, 102
Dandruff Rinse, 186
Dandruff-Control Treatments,
        183
dark circles, 110
dehydration, 168
deodorants, 269–71
    Botanical Deodorant, 271
    chlorophyll, 17
    Citrus Deodorant, 271
    Deodorant Powder, 235
    Natural Deodorant Cream, 270
deodorizer, baking soda as, 16
Desert Wonder Shampoo, 175
Diaper Cream, 293–94
diet, 109, 168
    effect on skin and hair, 6–7
    and nails, 201
dried kelp, 14
drugstores, 13, 14
dry brushing, 148–49
dry hair, conditioning packs for,
        180
dry skin, 32, 33, 47, 58, 61
    masks for, 99, 105
    men, 282
    oatmeal masks for, 98

Easy Soap Balls, 265
Effleurage, 216
egg yolk, 69, 99
eggs, 13, 20, 62
    Egg Shampoo, 174
    facials, 4
    hair care products, 174, 182
    henna enhancer, 189
    as mask, 106
Egyptian Henna Conditioning
        Treatment, 190
Elbow Cream, Oatmeal, 43
Electric Pre-shave, 280
Empress Josephene's Cleanser,
        34
emulsifiers, 61, 69
energy, 168
English Ivy Body Massage,
        149–50
environment
    effect on skin and hair, 7
epsom salts (magnesium sulfate),
        18
equipment, 6, 11–13
essences, 214
essential oils, 13, 14, 18, 168, 214
    in baby oil, 291
    for massage, 160
    in perfume, 263
eucalyptus (scent), 168
eucalyptus oil, 122
Evening Nail Oil, 206
exercise, 168
exfoliation, 141, 266
    dry lips, 122
    methods of, 144
    in shaving, 281
extracts and flavorings, 18
eye care, natural, 110
Eye Cream
    Super, 81
    Tropical, 82–83
Eye Gel, Cooling, 111
Eye Makeup Remover, Gentle, 37

eyebrows, 119
eyedropper, 12
eyelashes, 110

Face Paints, Fantasy, 298–99
facial masks
    see masks
facial scrubs, cleansing, 144
    for men, 281
facial treatments, 91–111
    Beauty Mayo, 94
    Salsa, 101
    steps in, 93
    see also cleansers; creams; masks
Fantasy Face Paints, 298–99
farmers' markets, 13, 14
fat, in making soap, 251
fatigue, 168
Favorite Cleansing Grains, 38–39
feet
    Athlete's-Foot Cure, 283
    Invigorating Foot Rub,
        282–83
    massage, 166
    Mustard Bath, 136
    powders, 227, 237
    Pumice Scrub for the, 44
    Zanzibar Foot Oil, 166
Fennel Seed and Honey Toner,
    52
filters, 12
Firming Neck Cream, 82
fixatives, 214
Fizzing Bath Bombs, 3, 135
Flavored Coconut Lip Gloss, 117
Floral Aloe Vera Gel, 77
flossing, 248
flower petals
    in massage oil, 165
flowers, 18
    in bath environment, 138
    in soap, 263, 264
Foaming Bath Salts, 136
Foot Oil, Zanzibar, 166

Foot Rub, Invigorating, 282–83
footbath(s)
    Mustard Bath, 136
fragrance, 213–24
    After-Bath Splash, 222
    Attar of Roses, 223
    Effleurage, 216
    Hungary Water, 217
    Lavender Linen Spray, 224
    Mona Lisa Voile, 220–21
Frangipani Lotion, Australian,
    68–69
French Green Clay, 100
Fresh Carrot Mask, 108
Fresh Strawberry Bath, 295
Fruit Gel Masks, 105
Fruit Powder, Carmen Miranda,
    236
Fuller's Earth, 100
funnel, 12

gardenia, 18
Gardenia Oil, 165
gel(s)
    Cooling Eye Gel, 111
    Floral Aloe Vera Gel, 77
    Refreshsing Leg Gel, 76
    see also hair gel
gelatin
    hair-care product, 190
    masks, 105
Gentle Eye Makeup Remover,
    37
geographical location
    and skin type, 61
geranium oil
    for athlete's foot, 283
geraniums, 234
    scent, 168
germs, 109
Gin Skin Tonic, 56
glycerine, 18–19, 214, 271, 280
    humectant, 260, 263
    Soap, 260–61, 264

grape seed oil, 19, 167
    Lotion, 74
Grapefruit Cleanser, 36
grapefruit juice
    as styling lotion, 191
grater, 11
Greek Cold Cream, Original,
    64–65
Green French clay, 14
Green Goddess Body Mask, 151
green tea, 19
    Skin Toner, 3, 53
grocery stores, 13, 14
gums, brushing, 241
Gyokura, 19

hair
    covering in sunlight, 154
    factors affecting, 6–7
    henna for, 19
hair care, 171
    swimming pool, 197
hair-care products, 171–97
    Brilliantine, 193
    Dandruff-Control Treatments,
        183
    for men, 284, 285, 286
    see also hair color; hair
        conditioners; hair gel; hair
        rinses; hair styling aids;
        shampoos
hair color
    henna enhancers, 189
    Henna, 187–88
hair conditioners, 21, 171
    Caribbean Rum, 182
    Egyptian Henna Conditioning
        Treatment, 190
    grape seed oil, 19
    Perfect Hair, 181
    Roaring Twenties, 182
    Rock Melon, 181
    Tucson Jojoba Oil and Beer,
        182

hair gel
  Almond Oil, 192
  Basic, 190–91
  Champagne, 193
  Pink Grapefruit Styling Gel,
    191
hair growth products, 19, 194
hair oil(s)
  Brilliantine, 193
  Rosemary, 194
Hair Packs
  Avocado Oil, 284
  conditioning, 179–80
  Honey (Molasses), 180
hair rinses, 171
  beer as, 16
  Dandruff Rinse, 186
  highlighting (list), 185
  lemon juice as, 20
  natural (list), 184
  Watercress Rinse for Oily
    Hair, 186
hair setting lotion, beer as, 16
Hair Spray
  Lemon, 195
  Sugar, 196
hair styling aids, 171
  Champagne Hair Gel, 193
  grape seed oil as, 19
  Pink Grapefruit Styling Gel,
    191
  Psyllium-Seed Setting Lotion,
    196
  tools, 192
Hair Tonic, Jalapeño, 194–95
Hair Treatment, Horseradish, 285
hand care/hands, 201
  hot wax treatments, 209
  manicure, 202–3
  mask, 203
  Paraffin Hand Treatment, 209
  Pumice Hand Scrub, 284
Hand Scrub, Pumice, 284
Hand Treatment, Paraffin, 209

hand mixer/electric whisk, 12
Health Nut Lotion, 76–77
heat rash, 238
Helen of Troy, 5, 125
Henna
  Egyptian Henna Conditioning
    Treatment, 190
  Enhancers, 189
  Hair Color, 187–88
  leaves, 19
  Mehndi-Henna Tattoos,
    152–53
  Nail Treatment, 207
Herb shop, 14
herbs
  exotic, 14
  herb baths, 129–30
  Herb Garden Mouthwash,
    242
  Herb Massage Oil, 162
  Herbal Body Wrap, 145
  Herbal Shampoo, 174
  mouthwash, 242
  relaxing, 162
  in soaps, 264
  stimulating, 162
  teas, 19
  Vinegar-Herb Bath, 127–28
heredity
  effect on skin and hair, 7
hibiscus flowers
  hair rinse, 185
highlighting hair rinses (list), 185
Hippocrates, 125
Honey, 19–20, 99
  Bee Bath, 295
  as cleanser, 32
  Cleanser, All-Purpose, 34
  Fennel Seed and Toner, 52
  (Molasses) Hair Pack, 180
  Toner, 5, 51
Horseradish Hair Treatment, 285
Hot Rock Massage, 163
hot wax treatments, 209

humectant
  glycerine, 260, 263
  honey, 20, 51
  molasses, 205
Hungary Water, 217
hydrotherapy, 125–38

indigestion, 18
ingredients, 4, 5
  basic, 15–26
  optional, 7, 8
  shopping for, 13–15
Invigorating Foot Rub, 282–83
iodine, 109, 146
Irish moss, 85
iron, 21, 98
Irresistible Rose Cologne, 218

Jalapeño Hair Tonic, 194–95
jars, 13
jojoba bean oil, 20
Jojoba Nail and Cuticle Oil, 204
Jojoba Oil, Tucson, and Beer
    Conditioner, 182

Kaolin Clay, 100
knives, 11

lactic acid, 32, 37
Langhorne, Irene, 224
lanolin, 13, 14, 20
Lanolin Cream, Australian,
    70–71
lavender, 18, 77, 162, 213
  Bath, Relaxing, 137
  Dry Perfume, 221
  effects of, 130
  Freshener, 57
  in hair care products, 174, 178,
    185
  Linen Spray, 224
  Mouth Rinse, 247
  in soap, 264
lavender oil, 55

lecithin, 99, 106, 182
   Moisturizer, 69–70
Leg Gel, Refreshing, 76
lemon juice, 20, 21, 32, 33
   in hair-care products, 176, 184
lemons, 20, 54
   Lemon Hair Spray, 195
   scent, 168
lighting
   in bath environment, 138
lip balm, 115
   Castor Oil, 119
Lip Gloss, 115
   Almond and Cocoa Butter, 116
   Aloe Vera, 116
   Chocolate, 3, 118
   Coconut-Almond, 117
   Flavored Coconut, 117
   Marie's Glitter Gloss, 298
   Tutti-Frutti, 297
   Vanilla, 118
lip paints, 115
Lip Stains, 120–21
lip treatments, 115–22
   Chapped Lip Cure, 121
lips, luscious, 122
lipstick, 115
   Beeswax, 119–20
liquid soap, 263
liquor stores, 14
Loofah Body Polish, 152
Loofah Soap, 266
Loofah (Luffa), sponge, 26–27,
   144
lotions, 61–87
   Alligator Pear, 80–81
   Allover Nighttime, 79–80
   Almond Oil, 67–68
   Australian Frangipani, 68–69
   Cooling Aloe, 78
   Corn Flour, 73
   Grape Seed Oil, 74
   Health Nut, 76–77
   for massage, 159, 160

   for men, 275, 280
   Mermaid, 85–86
   Mint Body, 84–85
   pre-shave, 280
   Rose, 87
   Witch Hazel Body, 78–79
   Yarrow, 83–84
lye
   in making soap, 251

macadamia nut oil, 4, 20
magnesium, 21, 98
manicure, 4, 202–3
Marie Antoinette, 5, 95
Marie Antoinette Mask, 95
Marie's Glitter Gloss, 298
marigold (calendula), 18, 77
marjoram
   effects of, 130
Mary, Queen of Scots, 125
masks, 4, 91, 203
   Apricot Facial, 96
   avocados, 16
   Beauty Queen, 99
   Brewer's Yeast, 104
   Country Garden Facial, 96
   Fresh Carrot, 108
   Fruit Gel, 105
   Marie Antoinette Mask, 95
   Mediterranean, 102
   Natural Clay, 99–100
   Old-Fashioned Oatmeal, 98
   Piña Colada, 107
   single-ingredient, 106–7
   Strawberry Acne, 108
   Summer Watermelon, 101
   Surprise-Party Facial, 97
   Swedish Rose Hip, 103
   Swiss Milkmaid, 102
   see also Body Mask
massage, 159
   avocado pits in, 27
   baby, 291–92
   foot, 166

   Hot Rock, 163
   how to give, 160
massage oils, 19, 159–68
   Amorous, 161
   Citrus, 163
   Cooling Massage Spirits, 166
   for feet, 283
   Gardenia Oil, 165
   Herb, 162
   Oil of Oils, 164
   Sore Muscle, 164
   Vintage Oil, 167
   Zanzibar Foot Oil, 166
mayonnaise, 13, 15, 20–21
   in beauty treatments, 94
   hair pack, 179
   as mask, 106
measuring cups and spoons, 11,
   12
medication
   effect on skin and hair, 7
Mediterranean Mask, 102
Mehndi-Henna Tattoos, 152–53
men, products for, 275–86
   Avocado Oil Hair Pack, 284
   cleansing facial scrubs, 281
   Crew-Cut Oil, 286
   Electric Pre-shave, 280
   Horseradish Hair Treatment,
   285
   Moustache Wax, 285
   Pumice Hand Scrub, 284
   Scrubbing Sacks, 134
   Vitalizing Skin Bracer, 279
menthol, 50
Mermaid Lotion, 85–86
microwave oven, 13
milk
   as cleanser, 32, 37
   Cleansing Milk, 33
milk baths, 125
   Cleopatra, 128
   New Baby Bath, 294
mineral oil, 14, 21

minerals, 104
minifacial, 93
mink oil, 22
mint, 162
    Body Lotion, 84–85
    effects of, 130
    leaves, 50
    in soap, 264
    -Vinegar Toner, 52
moisturizer(s), 16, 21, 31, 61
    Basic, 71–72
    Lecithin, 69–70
Molasses Nail Soak, 205
Mona Lisa Voile, 220–21
mood, scents and, 159
Morning Wake-up!, 126
Moustache Wax, 285
mouth fresheners, natural, 244
mouthwashes, 241–48
    Clove, 243
    Herb Garden, 242
    Lavender Mouth Rinse, 247
    Rose Water, 242
    Salt Water Rinse, 245
    Strawberry Leaf Mouth Rinse,
       243–44
Muscle-Soothing Bath, Super,
    129
musk, 161, 213, 214
Mustard Bath, 136

Nail Hardener, 207
nail polish, 202
    Natural, 205
nail polish remover, 202
nail treatments, 201–9
    Caster Oil Nail Rub, 208
    Cocoa Cuticle Cream, 204
    Evening Nail Oil, 206
    Henna Nail Treatment, 207
    Jojoba Nail and Cuticle Oil,
       204
    Molasses Nail Soak, 205
    Nail Hardener, 207

Nail Whitener, 208
    Natural Nail Polish, 205
    Pineapple Cuticle Softener,
       206
Nail Whitener, 208
nails
    care of, 201–2
    henna for, 19
    manicure, 202–3
    polishing, 202, 203
natural beauty, 3–6
    ten steps to, 6
natural beauty products
    care and storage guidelines, 8
    cost savings, 5
    recipes, 3, 4, 5–6, 7–8
    see also ingredients
natural beauty tools, 26–28
Natural Clay Masks, 99–100
Natural Deodorant Cream, 270
natural fat, 32
natural food stores, 13, 14
natural hair rinses (list), 184
natural mouth fresheners, 244
Natural Nail Polish, 205
natural oils, 16, 23
    as lip treatment, 115
Neck Cream, Firming, 82
nectarine pits, 41
Nefertiti, 221, 224
New Baby Bath, 294
normal hair
    conditioning packs for, 180
normal skin, 58, 61
    masks for, 105
    oatmeal masks for, 98
Northwest Pine Bath, 130–31

oatmeal, 21
    in bath, 297
    cleanser, 31, 32, 33
    Cleanser, 33
    Cookie Bath, 132
    Elbow Cream, 43

    for facial scrub, 144
    Old-Fashioned Oatmeal
       Masks, 98
    scrubs, 4
    Soap, 259–60
    Soap, Super-Easy, 262
oil(s), 20
    Baby Oil, 291
    Coconut Baby Oil, 293
    in creams and lotions, 61, 62
    massage, 159, 160
    see also specific types of oils
Oil of Oils, 164
oily hair
    conditioning packs for, 180
    Watercress Rinse for, 186
oily skin, 32, 36, 47, 49, 58, 61,
    143
    masks for, 105
    oatmeal masks for, 98
Old West Aftershave, 278
Old-Fashioned Bubble Bath,
    133
Old-Fashioned Oatmeal Masks,
    98
olive oil, 21
    Cleansing Lotion, 35
    Shampoo, 176
orange and lime peel
    ground dried, in facial scrub,
       281
orange flower water, 21
orange oil (neroli), 21, 233
Orange Peel Scrub, 39–40
Orange-Flower Powder, 233
Orange-Mint Toner, 50
Orchid Isle Cologne, 219
oregano, 162
Original Greek Cold Cream,
    64–65
orrisroot
    in powder, 230, 234
orrisroot powder, 21–22, 214
    dry shampoo, 177

pans, 12
pansy, 18
papain, 75
Papaya Cream, 75
Paraffin Hand Treatment, 209
patchouli, 18
peach pits, 41
pear
   as mask, 107
pear juice, 49
pectin, 49
pedicures, 4, 202
peelers, 11
peppermint, 18, 122, 213
   oil, 84, 126
   Powder, 232
   scent, 168
   Toothpaste, 247
Perfect Hair Conditioner, 181
Perfume(s), 213, 214
   Citrus Dry, 222
   dry, 221, 222
   Lavender Dry, 221
   soap, 263
   Solid, 224
petroleum jelly, 21
pharmacies, 14, 15
phosphates, 21, 98
physical activity
   effect on skin and hair, 7
Piesse, Septimus, 213
Piña Colada Mask, 107
Pine Bath, Northwest, 130–31
Pineapple, 107
   Body Seltzer, 126–27
   Cuticle Softener, 206
Pink Grapefruit Styling Gel,
   191
Play Dough, Scented, 299
Pompadour, Madame de, 224
potassium, 21, 98
   in honey, 19
Potpourris, 22
pots, enamel or steel, 252

Powder, 227–38
   Almond Oil, 231
   Baby, 290
   Carmen Miranda Fruit, 236
   Chlorophyll, 228
   Cloud Nine, 237
   Cooling Cinnamon, 238
   Deodorant, 235
   Orange-Flower, 233
   Peppermint, 232
   Rose Geranium, 234
   Scented Bath, 229
   Scented Rice Flour, 230
   Simple Bath, 228, 230
   Violet, 234
   see also tooth powders
powdered orange peel
   as tooth powder, 246
preservatives, 7–8
   aspirin, 16
   lecithin, 99
   tincture of benzoin, 23
   vitamin C, 23, 54
prevention, 109
   of wrinkles, 110
protein, 16, 21, 32, 98, 102, 106,
      132, 146, 182, 191, 193
   for nails, 201
Psyllium-Seed Setting Lotion,
   196
puffiness, under-eye, 110
Pumice
   Hand Scrub, 284
   Scrub for the Feet, 44
pumice stone, 27, 144

Raw Sugar Scrub, 143
Refreshing Leg Gel, 76
refrigeration, 8, 92, 141
relaxation
   body treatments in, 141
Relaxing Lavender Bath, 137
rest, 109
Rhassoul Mud, 100

rhubarb
   hair rinse, 185
Rice Flour
   Dry Shampoo, 178
   Powder, Scented, 230
   in powders, 227
Roaring Twenties Conditioner,
   182
Rock Melon Hair Conditioner,
   181
Roman Empire Aftershave,
   278–79
rose, 18
   Attar of Roses, 223
   Floral Bath, 131
   Irresistible Rose Cologne,
      218
   Lotion, 87
   scent, 161
Rose Geranium
   Powder, 234
   soap, 263
rose hips, 54
   Swedish Rose Hip Mask, 103
rose petals
   in soap, 264
rose water, 13, 14, 19, 22
   Mouthwash, 242
rosemary, 162
   effects of, 130
   Hair Oil, 194
   scent, 168
   in shampoo, 174, 178
Rough skin areas, 31, 75, 144
   Oatmeal Elbow Cream, 43
rubber gloves, 252
Rum, Caribbean, Conditioner,
   183

saffron, 263
sage
   effects of, 130
   hair rinse, 185
   tooth powder, 246

salicylic acid
  see aspirin (salicylic acid)
Salsa Facial, 101
salt (sodium chloride), 13, 22
  dry shampoo, 177
  rubs, 144
  Salt Rub, 142
  as tooth powder, 245–46
Salt Water Rinse, 245
sand, 28
  as scrub, 44
sandalwood, 18, 213
  scent, 161
saponification, 22, 251–52
scent groups, 213–14
  list, 214
Scented Bath Powder, 229
Scented Play Dough, 299
Scented Rice Flour Powder, 230
scents, 7, 159, 168, 213, 214–15
  children's products, 289
  essential oils, 18
  layering, 216
  for men, 275
  solid, 224
Scrubbing Sacks, 134
scrubs, 23, 31, 38–44, 109
  Almond Cleansing, 38
  Apricot Kernel, 41
  Avocado Stone, 40–41
  body, 152
  facial, 144, 281
  Favorite Cleansing Grains,
    38–39
  Loofah Body Polish, 152
  oatmeal, 4, 144
  Oatmeal Elbow Cream, 43
  Orange Peel, 39–40
  Pumice, for the Feet, 44
  Pumice Hand Scrub, 284
  Raw Sugar, 143
  Sublime Sunflower, 42
  Sugar, 43
Sea Mud Body Mask, 145–46

sea sponge, 27
seawater treatments, 146
seaweed, 85
semolina flour
  dry shampoo, 177
sense of smell, 159, 213
sensitive skin, 32, 33, 82
  Astringent for, 48
  oatmeal masks, 98
sesame oil, 22, 73
shampoos, 22, 172
  Basic Shampoo A, 173
  Basic Shampoo B, 173
  Basil Shampoo Powder, 178
  Body and Bounce, 175
  Desert Wonder, 175
  dry, 177, 178
  Egg, 174
  Herbal, 174
  Olive Oil, 176
  Rice Flour Dry, 178
  Sunshine, 176
  tips for, 171–72
shaving, 281
shaving creams, 275
  Almond Oil, 282
  Basic, 280–81
shaving tips, 275–76
shower
  following dry brushing, 148
  hot/cold, 125
shower treatments, 125–38
  Morning Wake-up!, 126
  Pineapple Body Seltzer,
    126–27
silicon, 21, 98
Simple Bath Powder, 228, 230
skin, 20, 109, 144
  children, 289
  clean, healthy, 91, 109
  factors affecting, 6–7
  functions of, 141
  zinc oxide healing, 26
Skin Bracer, Vitalizing, 279

skin freshener, 47, 55–57
  Beauty Water, 57
  Chamomile, 55–56
  Citrus, 55
  Gin Skin Tonic, 56
  Lavender, 57
  witch hazel, 24
skin softener
  cocoa butter, 17
Skin Toner, Green Tea, 3, 53
skin type, 32, 61
  one-minute test, 58
  testing, 61
skin-softening routines, 125
sleep, 168
smile, healthy, 248
smoking, 110
soap, 4–5, 22, 31, 251–66
  Basic Castile, 255–56
  castile, 13, 17, 262
  Coconut Oil, 256–57
  Cold-Cream, 258–59
  colored, 263
  Easy Soap Balls, 265
  Glycerine, 260–61
  liquid, 263
  Loofah, 266
  natural alternatives, 32
  Oatmeal, 259–60
  perfume, 263
  Soap Treasures, 264–65
  Super-Easy Oatmeal, 262
  Tallow, 254–55
Soap Balls, Easy, 265
soap making, 251–56
  equipment (list), 252
  ingredient temperatures, 253
  rules, 253
  variations in, 263–64
soap molds, 252
Soap Treasures, 264–65
sodium hydroxide, 251
Solid Perfume, 224
Soothing Aftershave, 277

Soothing Tooth Powder, 246
Sore Muscle Massage Oil, 164
sore muscles, 18
sound
    in bath environment, 138
sour cream, 32
soy lecithin, 69
specialty stores, 14
spice
    henna enhancer, 189
spot test
    new products/treatments, 8
steaming, 109
stearic acid, 22, 71
stearic acid powder, 14
stirring rod, 12
strainer, 12
stove/hot plate/electric skillet, 13
strawberries
    as mask, 106
Strawberry
    Acne Mask, 108
    Cleanser, 36
Strawberry Leaf
    Astringent, 49
    Mouth Rinse, 243–44
Stretch Mark Cream, 86
Sublime Sunflower Scrub, 42
substitutions, 25
sugar
    as cleanser, 32
    facial scrub, 144
    Hair Spray, 196
    Raw Sugar Scrub, 143
    Scrub, 43
sugarbrasion, 43
Summer Garden Cologne, 220
Summer Watermelon Mask, 101
sun, 154
sun protection
    on lips, 115
sunblock
    zinc oxide, 26
Sunburn Soothers, 155

Sunflower, Sublime, Scrub, 42
sunflower seeds, 23
    ground, in facial scrub, 281
sunglasses, 110, 154
sunscreen, 61, 154
    on lips, 122
Sunshine Shampoo, 176
Super Eye Cream, 81
Super Muscle-Soothing Bath, 129
Super-Easy Oatmeal Soap, 262
superstores, 14
Surprise-Party Facial Mask, 97
Swedish Rose Hip Mask, 103
sweet birch leaves, 16
Sweet Dreams Bath, 297
Swimming Pool Hair Care,
    197
Swiss Milkmaid Mask, 102, 203

talc, 227, 290
tallow, 251
    Soap, 254–55
tea bags, 19
tea tree oil, 23
teas
    henna enhancer, 189
    herbal, 19
teeth
    brushing, 241, 245, 248
tetracycline, 7
thalassotherapy, 146
thickening agent(s)
    cornstarch, 18
tincture of benzoin, 8, 23
tomato
    as mask, 107
tomato juice
    hair rinse, 184
toners, 47, 50–52
    Cooling Cucumber, 51
    Fennel Seed and Honey, 52
    Green Tea Skin, 53
    Honey, 51
    Mint-Vinegar, 52

Orange-Mint, 50
    Vitamin C, 54
tooth powders, 241–48
    baking soda, 16
    Soothing Tooth Powder, 246
Toothpaste, Peppermint, 247
toxins, 149
Tropical Body Polish, 147
Tropical Eye Cream, 82–83
troubled skin care, 109
Tucson Jojoba Oil and Beer
        Conditioner, 182
turmeric, 263
Tutti-Frutti Lip Gloss, 297

United States Pharmacopeia
    (U.S.P.), 26, 279

vaginal yeast infections, 127
vanilla, 213
    Lip Gloss, 118
    in perfumes, 219
vegetable oils, 13, 71, 251
Victorian Handkerchief Cologne,
        218
vinegar (acetic acid), 13, 16,
        20–21, 23
    henna enhancer, 189
    -Herb Bath, 127–28
    Mint-Vinegar Toner, 52
vinotherapy, 167
Vintage Oil, 167
Violet Powder, 234
Vitalizing Skin Bracer, 279
Vitamin A, 16, 23, 24, 36, 96, 101,
        108
    for acne, 109
vitamin B, 16, 101, 104, 132
vitamin B_6
    for acne, 109
vitamin C (ascorbic acid), 8,
        23–24, 36, 49, 53, 101,
        103
Vitamin C Toner, 54

vitamin D, 154
vitamin E (tocopherol), 16, 23, 24, 53, 76, 78
vitamin E oil, 21, 42, 81
vitamin/mineral supplement, 109
vitamin shops, 14
vitamins, 102, 106
vodka (alcohol), 24
volatile oils, 214, 223

water, 13, 24, 109, 168, 171
  Beauty Water, 57
  in creams and lotions, 61
  for healing, 125
  as skin freshener, 47
Watercress Rinse for Oily Hair, 186
Watermelon Mask, Summer, 101
weights and measures, 28
wheat germ oil, 24, 76
wintergreen, 16
witch hazel (*hamamelis virginiana*), 13, 14, 24–26, 271
  in aftershave, 277
  Body Lotion, 78–79

wooden spoons, 252
World Wide Web/Internet, 14–15
wrinkles, 52, 110

Yarrow Lotion, 83–84
yogurt, 13, 15, 26, 31
  Body Treatment, 147
  as cleanser, 32, 33
  henna enhancer, 189
  as mask, 106

Zanzibar Foot Oil, 166
zinc, 109
zinc oxide, 26

About the Author

JANICE COX is America's leading home beauty expert who has been making her own beauty products and treatments for almost thirty years. Many of her recipes have been passed down through three generations of her family. She is the author of three books on natural beauty and writes for a number of national magazines and newspapers. Janice lives in Medford, Oregon, with her husband and two daughters.